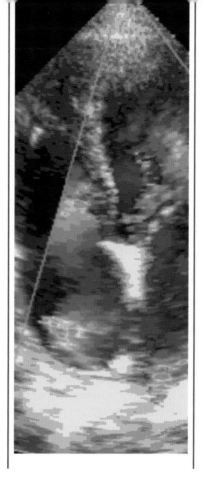

Cardio-Oncology
Case Study

Coordinators

Juan Carlos Plana
Teresa López Fernández
José Juan Gómez de Diego
Miguel Ángel García Fernández

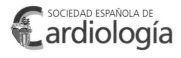

SOCIEDAD ESPAÑOLA DE
Cardiología

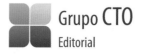

Grupo CTO
Editorial

DISCLAIMER

Medicine is a science subject to constant change. As research and clinical experience widen our knowledge, treatments and pharmacotherapy changes are necessary. The editors of this work have verified their results against reliable sources, in an effort to provide general and complete information, according to the accepted criteria at the time of publication. Nevertheless, given the fact that human error may occur or that some changes may take place in medical sciences, neither the editor nor any of the contributors involved in the preparation –or publication- of this work can guarantee that the content herein is accurate and complete in each and every aspect. The editors and the contributing sources cannot be held responsible for any errors, omissions or the outcome derived from the use of the information provided herein. Therefore, readers are recommended to verify the content of this work against other sources. As an example, it is especially advisable to read the package insert of any drug to be administered to ensure that the information furnished by this publication is accurate and no modifications were made either to the recommended dose or to the contraindications for administering said drug. This recommendation is particularly significant in relation to new or seldom used drugs. Readers should also check with their own laboratory about normal values.

© Sociedad Española de Cardiología, 2015. SEC: 2015-B
© CTO EDITORIAL, S.L. 2015

Edition, design and layout: CTO Editorial

C/ Francisco Silvela, 106; 28002 Madrid
Tel.: (0034) 91 782 43 30 - Fax: (0034) 91 782 43 43
E-mail: ctoeditorial@ctomedicina.com
Web Page: www.grupocto.es

ISBN Obra Completa: 978-84-16403-59-2
ISBN Cardio-Oncology Case Study: 978-84-16403-85-1
Legal Deposit: M-19653-2015

Printed in Spain - Impreso en España

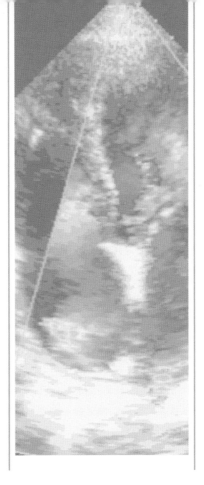

Cardio-Oncology
Case Study

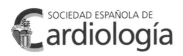

SOCIEDAD ESPAÑOLA DE
Cardiología

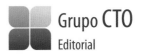

Grupo CTO
Editorial

Prologue

Cancer and cardiovascular disease share common features. First, the high rate of incidence of both pathologies. Second, they have several risk factors in common. Moreover, the treatment of both diseases has seen spectacular progress in the last few years and this, which is without a doubt positive, has a downside that is little mentioned: the sequelae of survival.

It is precisely this connection, the undesired common ground between cancer and cardiovascular diseases that has motivated the drawing up and publication of this book and the development of a specialty which, without a doubt, will give us a lot to talk about in the future: cardio-oncology.

We observed as early as the 1960s, when we started to predict that a battle against cancer could be waged successfully, that the introduction of a new therapeutic weapon against malignant tumors, anthracyclines, was accompanied by secondary cardiac dysfunction associated with the treatment.

Everything entails priorities and, in spite of this information, the effect was relegated to a second level; the important thing was to increase the rates of survival and for patients to live longer; quality of life was considered secondary until only recently.

The situation is different now and cancer is cured in a higher percentage of cases (which can be very high according to kind of tumor). We therefore find ourselves faced with a pool of patients who, without actually being named in this way, act as such in part because of the sequelae of the chemotherapy, among these cardiovascular toxicity. These are people who, in addition to having suffered from cancer, in many cases have the only non-modifiable risk factor for cardiovascular disease, which is age. For this reason, their cardiology treatment is a top priority.

Against this backdrop, I think it is an excellent idea to come to an agreement on multidisciplinary management of cancer patients that includes cardiovascular care and, especially notable, the project outlined here on the creation of cardio-oncology units.

It is time to put an end to the perception that toxicity because of cancer treatment is an irreversible situation and this is manifested as such in this book. I hope this reaches all professionals who, in one way or another, are involved in the battle against cancer and cardiovascular disease management.

Valentín Fuster
General Director *"Centro Nacional de Investigaciones Cardiovasculares Carlos III"* (CNIC) and Director of the Cardiovascular Institute. Madrid. Spain Physician-in-Chief, Mount Sinai Medical Center. New York. USA

Preface

Cardiovascular disease in patients with cancer and cardiac complications of cancer therapy: State of a new clinical art.

Cardiovascular diseases remain the main cause of mortality and morbidity worldwide and despite major advances on its management, these numbers will persist according to all the projections. On the other hand, malignancy also plays a significant role in the modern world, also related with ageing populations.

Tremendous advances in oncology treatments have occurred over the recent years which enabled to increase the life spam of some of these patients. However many of these medications have toxic effects, including, many of them, cardiotoxicity. Cardiotoxicity, revealed as a compromise in cardiac physiology, is, therefore, a major concern in cancer therapy. Breast cancer treatments, as an example, are especially prone to produce cardiotoxic effects, but not only the classical chemo and radiotherapies, also those based in specific blocking of receptors with monoclonal antibodies. The therapeutic approach to these patients include drugs with established potential cardiotoxicity, such as anthracyclines, but also new agents, namely trastuzumab, that has been shown to be associated with ventricular dysfunction. This points out the need of a strategy for early diagnosis of cardiotoxicity. Furthermore in a large number of breast cancer patients undergoing radiotherapy, the cardiac impact of actual techniques, particularly the cumulative effect of left breast irradiation and new chemotherapy drugs, remain uncertain. International guidelines recommend regular monitoring of cardiac function, especially through assessment of left ventricular ejection fraction, in patients treated with cardiotoxic agents. However, a decline of LVEF represents a relatively late stage on cardiac dysfunction when the damage to the myocardium has already been too extensive with less likelihood of recovery.

As a consequence, cardiotoxic effects can prevent the continuation of antitumoral treatments and for this reason, there is an urgent medical need to find reliable biomarkers of induced cardiotoxicity, including imaging parameters. From a histological point of view, cardiotoxicity induced by anthracyclines, the most studied agents, is characterized mainly by necrosis. Thus, the role of biomarkers of myocardial necrosis has been studied by different groups. Troponin I (TnI) has high sensitivity (> 90%) yet low specificity (71%) to predict ventricular ejection fraction impairment after anthracycline administration. However, the first biomarker to be described, B-type natriuretic peptide (BNP) and its N-terminal pro-fragment (NT-proBNP) are well established predictors of adverse outcome in heart failure and acute coronary syndrome. Although some results are conflicting, there seems to be a trend showing an elevation of BNP after chemotherapy and an association with ventricular dysfunction. However, its role in risk stratification needs to be further assessed.

In recent years, a few researchers have investigated the role of gene expression on cardiotoxicity mainly related to doxorubicin chemotherapy. Several potential candidate genomic biomarkers for cardiotoxicity have been identified in rats by microarray analysis. MiRNAs are small non-coding RNAs that act at the post-transcriptional level regulating the protein output and miRNA stability. Some miRNAs have been described as crucial elements in the development and function in the cardiac system. Several studies have shown that miRNAs can modulate a diverse spectrum of cardiac functions with developmental, physiological, and clinical implications. MiRNA expression patterns are altered in both human and in animal models of cardiac disease. Modulation of miRNA expression in vitro and in vivo has revealed the important role of miRNAs in regulating heart function, particularly cardiac growth and conductance. Differential expression of miRNAs seems to play an important role in the development of chemotherapy induced cardiotoxicity. Some specific miRNAs are actively secreted by cells, constituting a possible way of cell-to-cell communication. Circulating miRNAs in plasma or serum were postulated as clinical biomarkers of several cardiovascular conditions.

This is one important area of research that may translate into potential clinical applications for the early identification of cardiotoxicity, therefore, helping in tailoring the treatment in these patients.

Malignancy itself induces changes in the normal homeostasis with potential major implications in the development of disease processes, which may be systemic, but many times involving the cardiovascular system, such as the case of vascular phenomenon as well as cardiac manifestations (heart failure, dysrhythmias, pericarditis, among others). In some cases the cardiovascular involvement by the malignant process may actually represent its main expression.

In accordance to these findings, the field of the so called cardio-oncology has grown fast over the last few years. This implies the need to develop proper educational tools that can help to educate and train the medical community. This is why the current textbook is so relevant since it is one of the first to address specifically the issue of cardio-oncology.

I have to congratulate the Spanish Society of Cardiology for the initiative which fills-in an unmet need until now. In this textbook all the main issues related with cardio-oncology are addressed in a very practical way and at the same time with an indepth review of the main current topics. Some of the main players in the field, mostly from the Spanish cardiological community, have contributed to this project. Therefore, I also agree this may represent for our community a state of a new clinical art involving a very special group of patients, the oncology patients. At the same time it is an excellent example on how different medical specialities can, and should, work together. I am sure this will be another milestone in the combat against cardiovascular disease which is our main mission as scientific-medical cardiological community.

Lisbon, May 2015.

Fausto J. Pinto
President of the European Society of Cardiology
University Hospital Santa Maria
University of Lisbon, Portugal

Preamble

Cardiovascular disease and cancer are the leading determining factors of mortality, quality of life and health costs in the vast majority of countries. The increasing survival of cancer patients has created new needs in the social and healthcare network. Cardiovascular involvement in cancer patients is an emergent discipline in medicine. Cancer as a systemic disease has a variety of acute and chronic harmful effects on the structure and function of the heart and its associated vessels. However, the multimodal treatment strategy frequently used for cancer treatment radiotherapy cytostatic drugs, etc. often has a direct toxic effect on the cardiovascular system. The multidisciplinary approach required to wage the modern battle against cancer should include strategies for cardiovascular assessment in patients with cancer and, most importantly, to avoid acute and chronic cardiovascular disease in this important and increasing group of patients. Therefore, the relationship between cardiologists and oncologists is a priority in the health system to plan the optimal care of cancer patients; this is needed above all to organize patient evaluations including the assessment of global cardiovascular risk including classical risk factors and lifestyle changes such as stopping smoking, dietary habits, physical exercise, etc., and other risk factors such as hypertension, diabetes, lipid disorders, etc. Imaging techniques play a critical role in functional and structural cardiac and vascular evaluation prior to cancer treatment and in follow-up to detect early changes that need specific therapy or influence cancer therapy.

This new book of the Spanish Society of Cardiology library is probably the first compendium from a clinical point of view of all the aspects that should be taken into account when planning cancer patient care. I am convinced this will be of major value for all healthcare professionals involved in the care of patients with cancer.

José Ramón González Juanatey
President of the Spanish Society of Cardiology

Foreword

Evolving cardiovascular care strategies have identified teamwork as the core of modern oncology. The Cardio-Oncology clinical cases atlas is intended as a starting point to organize multidisciplinary care of cancer patients. By means of 20 clinical cases, we gather practical information about diagnosis, management and prevention of cancer therapeutic-related cardiac diseases. The two major goals are minimize cancer treatment interruptions and ensure long-term event-free cardiovascular survival.

Aware of the importance of cardiac imaging techniques for cardiotoxicity diagnosis, this book is printed with the application of augmented reality, which enables reproducing the videos printed inside on an electronic device.

This project would not have been possible without the support of the Spanish Society of Cardiology. We thank all the authors for their work and dedication to the project, as well as CTO Editorial for all its efforts to ensure an attractive and pioneering work.

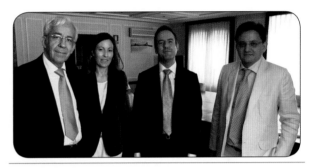

Video presentation

Juan Carlos Plana

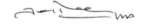

Teresa López Fernández

José Juan Gómez de Diego

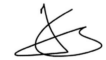

Miguel Ángel García Fernández

Coordinators

Juan Carlos Plana, MD, FACC, FASE
Chief of Clinical Operations
Don Chapman, MD Endowed Chair in Cardiology
Director Cardio-Oncology Center of Excellence
Associate Professor of Medicine. Section of Cardiology, Baylor College of Medicine. Houston. Texas. USA

Teresa López Fernández, MD
Cardiology Department. Cardiac Imaging Laboratory. La Paz University Hospital. IdiPaz Research Institute. Madrid. Spain

Juan José Gómez de Diego, MD
Cardiovascular Imaging Unit. San Carlos University Hospital. Madrid. Spain
Medicine Department. Complutense University of Madrid. Madrid. Spain
Teaching Director of the Spanish Association of Cardiac Imaging

Miguel Angel García Fernández, MD, PhD
Professor of Medicine. Complutense University of Madrid. Madrid. Spain
Cardiovascular Imaging Unit. San Carlos University Hospital. Madrid. Spain
General Secretary of the Spanish Society of Cardiology. President of the Spanish Association of Cardiac Imaging

Authors

Blázquez Bermejo, Zorba
Cardiology Department. La Paz University Hospital. IdiPaz Research Institute. Madrid. Spain

Caro Codón, Juan
Cardiology Department. La Paz University Hospital. IdiPaz Research Institute. Madrid. Spain

Cecconi, Alberto
Cardiology Department. San Carlos University Hospital. Madrid. Spain

Del Prado Díaz, Susana
Cardiology Department. La Paz University Hospital. IdiPaz Research Institute. Madrid. Spain

Ferrera Durán, Carlos
Cardiology Department. San Carlos University Hospital. Madrid. Spain

Freitas Ferraz, Afonso
Cardiology Department. San Carlos University Hospital. Madrid. Spain

Gómez de Diego, José Juan
Cardiology Department. San Carlos University Hospital. Madrid. Spain

González Fernández, Oscar
Cardiology Department. La Paz University Hospital. IdiPaz Research Institute. Madrid. Spain

López Fernández, Teresa
Cardiology Department. La Paz University Hospital. IdiPaz Research Institute. Madrid. Spain

Martínez Losas, Pedro
Cardiology Department. San Carlos University Hospital. Madrid. Spain

Olmos Blanco, Carmen
Cardiology Department. San Carlos University Hospital. Madrid. Spain

Rosillo Rodríguez, Sandra
Cardiology Department. La Paz University Hospital. IdiPaz Research Institute. Madrid. Spain

Valbuena López, Silvia
Cardiology Department. La Paz University Hospital. IdiPaz Research Institute. Madrid. Spain

Content

CASE STUDY

Index

Cardio-Oncology
Case Study

Case 01

Chronic Anthracycline-Induced Cardiotoxicity

Teresa López Fernández*
José Juan Gómez de Diego**

* Cardiology Department. La Paz University Hospital. IdiPAz Research Institute. Madrid. Spain
** Cardiology Department. San Carlos University Hospital. Madrid. Spain

1.1. Case Presentation

A 44-year-old woman with a history of invasive ductal mamma carcinoma (pT1, cpN1a, G2, RH + HER2-) was admitted to the emergency department because of heart failure. The patient had been in her usual state of health until two months ago, when she reported progressive dyspnea, fatigue, abdominal distension, and peripheral edema. A total of 15 months before admission she had received combination chemotherapy with doxorubicin, cyclophosphamide and paclitaxel, followed by radiation therapy.

At the moment of presentation in the emergency department the patient complained of unease. She was alert and oriented. Her blood pressure was 100/50 mmHg; her heart rate was 110 bpm and her oxygen saturation was 91%. Auscultation revealed attenuated heart sounds with a pansystolic murmur (punctum maximum at the apex) and late inspiratory crackles audible over both lung fields. The ECG confirmed sinus tachycardia (110 bpm) with no associated repolarization abnormalities and the chest X-ray confirmed mild cardiomegaly and interstitial edema. Laboratory testing showed normal serum creatinine, NT-proBNP 32.560 pg/mL (normal range < 125 pg/mL), and TnI 0,25 ng/mL (normal range < 0,027 ng/mL). Upon diagnosis of acute heart failure, standard medical therapy was initiated.

Echocardiographic examination showed mild left ventricular dilatation (end diastolic volume 82 mL/m²) and global left ventricular hypokinesia with overall severely impaired systolic function (2D-ejection fraction 24% and 3D-ejection fraction 27%) (Video 1.1, Video 1.2, and Video 1.3). Left ventricle filling pressures were also increased (E/E'ratio at the lateral side of mitral annulus of 22).

A severe decrease in global longitudinal strain (GLS -5.6%) was documented (Video 1. 4), as well as a severe mitral regurgitation (Video 1.5, Video 1.6, and Figure 1.1). Right ventricular function was normal (TAPSE 17 mm; S´ 11.2 cm/s).

An echocardiogram performed eight months before, in order to rule out endocarditis, already revealed a mild reduction in left ventricular systolic function (end diastolic volume 75 mL/m²; 2D-Ejection Fraction 48%; E/E´ 12; MAPSE 10 mm) and a mild mitral regurgitation.

Heart failure treatment was commenced, and at seven-months follow-up we found an initial recovery in echo parameters: 2D-ejection fraction of 45% (Video 1.7) with a GLS of -13% (Figure 1.2) and mild mitral regurgitation (Video 1.8). However, despite improvements in systolic function the patient continued to experience exercise intolerance and was finally referred to a cardiac rehabilitation heart failure program, which consisted of specific exercise training and congestive heart failure self-care counseling. At one-year follow-up she remained in NYHA class I and on beta-blocker, ACEI and eplerenone treatment.

Videos

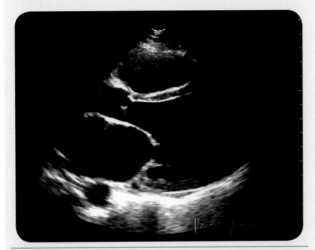

Video 1.1. 2D parasternal long-axis view of the left ventricle

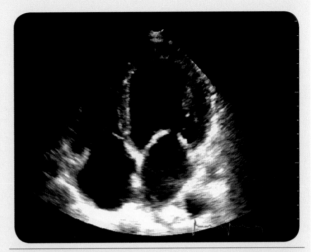

Video 1.2. 2D four-chamber view

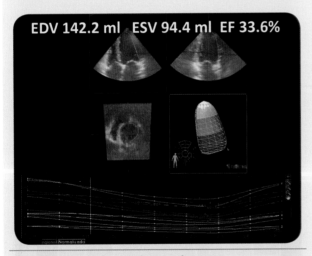

EDV 142.2 ml   ESV 94.4 ml   EF 33.6%

Video 1.3. 3D quantification of ejection fraction

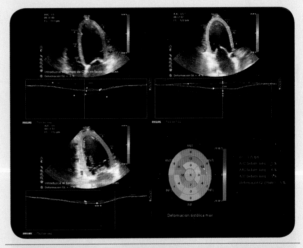

Video 1.4. Global longitudinal strain measurement

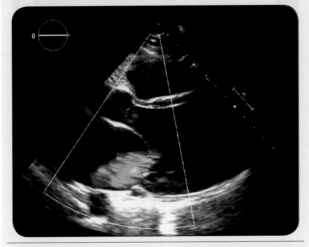

Video 1.5. 2D color severe mitral regurgitation

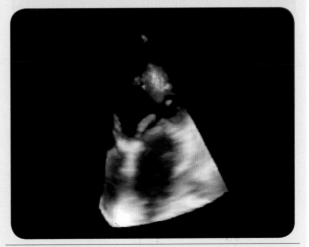

Video 1.6. 3D evaluation of mitral regurgitation

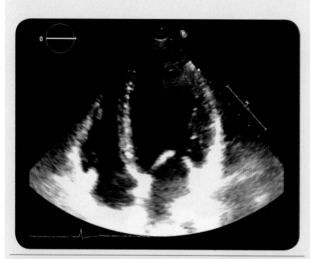

Video 1.7. Follow-up 2D-ejection fraction

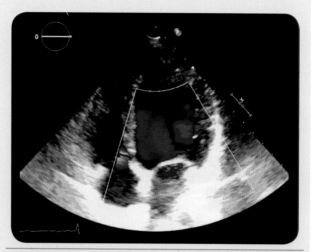

Video 1.8. 2D color mild mitral regurgitation

Figures

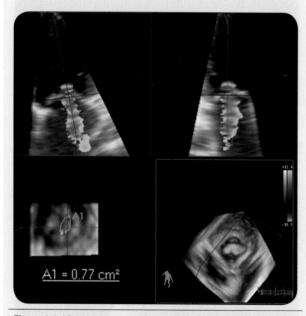

Figure 1.1. 3D vena contracta planimetry for quantification of mitral regurgitation severity

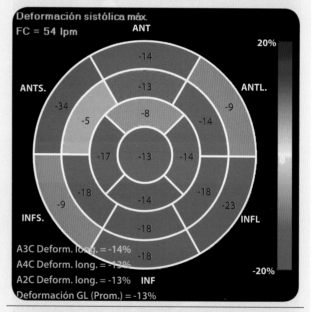

Figure 1.2. Follow-up global longitudinal strain

1.2. Discussion

Cardiovascular complications due to cardiotoxicity of chemotherapy are a growing problem that limits survival in cancer patients. Retrospectively it seemed that we had missed the opportunity to properly treat our patient. According to heart failure guidelines the diagnosis of an asymptomatic decrease in ejection fraction below 53% in a patient receiving chemotherapy must be classified as stage B heart failure. Thus, treatment is recommended in order to prevent left ventricular remodeling and symptoms. Since a timely initiation of adequate treatment is critical to maintain a patient's chances of recovery and depends on early diagnosis, cancer patients need to be monitored systematically.

A delay on initiation of heart failure treatment significantly reduces the chances of recovery of ventricular function. However, in the real world, many cancer patients with asymptomatic decrease in ejection fraction are not referred for cardiac consultation and do not receive proper heart failure treatment. In a recent study performed at Stanford University the vast majority of cancer patients with asymptomatic decrease in the ejection fraction did not receive cardiology consultation (Yoon GJ, *et al*. Left ventricular dysfunction in patients receiving cardiotoxic cancer therapies are clinicians responding optimally? *J Am Coll Cardiol* 2010; 56: 1.644-1.650). This suggests that closer collaboration between cardiologists and oncologists is needed to prevent and treat cardiovascular toxicity in cancer survivors.

Similar to other cardiac patients, cancer survivors are subject to the effects of deconditioning which eventually leads to a reduction in exercise tolerance. Cardiac rehabilitation programs through exercise training and heart failure self-care counseling confer significant clinical benefits on individuals with cardiotoxicity-related heart failure. Cardiac rehabilitation increases exercise capacity, improves clinical symptoms, enhances quality of life, and decreases future clinical events.

1.3. Conclusions

Cardiologists together with oncologists need to define criteria that help successfully identify high risk patients, introducing valuable and novel parameters (global longitudinal strain), so that therapeutic intervals are optimized.

Case 02

Subacute Anthracycline-Induced Cardiotoxicity

José Juan Gómez de Diego*
Teresa López Fernández**

* Cardiology Department. San Carlos University Hospital. Madrid. Spain
** Cardiology Department. La Paz University Hospital. IdiPAz Research Institute. Madrid. Spain

2.1. Case Presentation

A 79-year-old man with a history of non-Hodgkin's lymphoma (Diffuse large B-cell lymphoma IV A, IPI 4, aIPI 2) presented to the emergency department because of–sudden onset of dyspnea and hypotension. The patient had a previous history of type II diabetes and dyslipidemia treated only with diet; two months before admission he received chemotherapy for the lymphoma following the R-CHOP protocol (prednisone, vincristine, cyclophosphamide, doxorubicin, and rituximab) with achievement of full disease remission. ECG performed prior to chemotherapy was compatible with sinus rhythm and left bundle branch block. A baseline echocardiography showed a moderate dilated left atrium (left atrium indexed volume 43 mL/m^2), grade II diastolic dysfunction, and a 2D-ejection fraction of 57%.

On physical exam, the patient was diaphoretic with a blood pressure of 90/55 mmHg, body temperature of 36 °C, heart rate of 96 bpm, and an oxygen saturation of 100% maintained with a face mask with reservoir. The heart sounds were normal, with no murmurs. ECG this time showed atrial fibrillation with rapid ventricular rate and a left bundle branch block **(Figure 2.1).** An emergency echocardiography revealed a moderately dilated left ventricle with overall severely depressed systolic function,

a 2D-ejection fraction of 25% and grade III mitral regurgitation **(Video 2.1, Video 2.2, and Video 2.3).** The patient was transferred to the coronary unit, where he was started on non-invasive mechanical ventilation and concomitant heart failure drugs. After 12 hours, respiratory and hemodynamic stability were achieved. One week later, he was discharged on furosemide, carvedilol, losartan, digoxin, statins, and acenocumarol. Follow-up was scheduled as an outpatient for the progressive adjustment of heart failure therapy.

Six months after admission a follow-up echo showed mild left ventricular dysfunction with an end diastolic left ventricular volume of 88 mL/m^2, a 2D-ejection fraction of 49% and mild mitral regurgitation **(Video 2.4, Video 2.5, Video 2.6, and Video 2.7).** Global longitudinal strain was still affected (GLS -10.4%; **Figure 2.2).** The patient has had an uneventful clinical course with a NYHA functional class II under appropriate heart failure therapy. However, at two-year follow-up an asymptomatic decrease in ejection fraction was observed (3D-ejection fraction of 38%; **Video 2.8)** with a global longitudinal strain -6% **(Figure 2.3).** A cardiac magnetic resonance imaging (CMRI) confirmed this moderate decrease in left ventricular ejection fraction (EF 37%) and helped rule out the presence of perfusion defects or pathologic late gadolinium enhancement. Because of clinical stability no further investigation was performed.

Videos

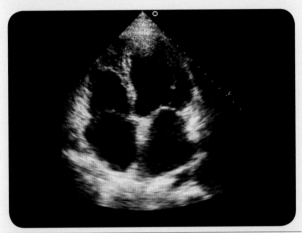

Video 2.1. 2D apical four-chamber view showed moderately dilated left ventricle with overall severely depressed systolic function

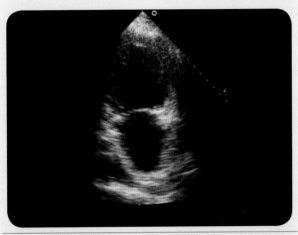

Video 2.2. 2D apical two-chamber apical view. 2D Simpson biplane ejection fraction was severely decreased (EF 25%)

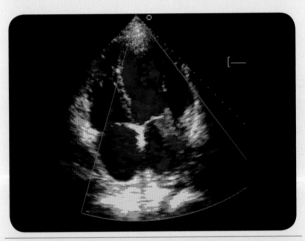

Video 2.3. 2D color apical four-chamber view showed significant mitral regurgitation secondary to left ventricular dilation

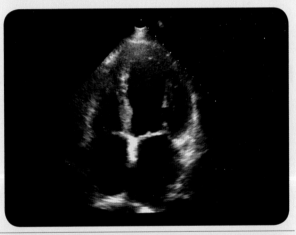

Video 2.4. 2D apical four-chamber view. Follow-up echocardiography performed on heart failure treatment and well controlled atrial fibrillation

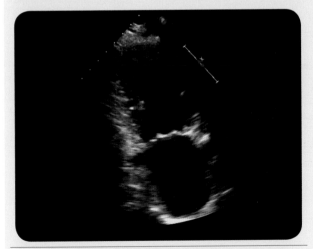

Video 2.5. 2D apical two-chamber apical view. 2D Simpson biplane ejection fraction was mildly decreased (EF 49%)

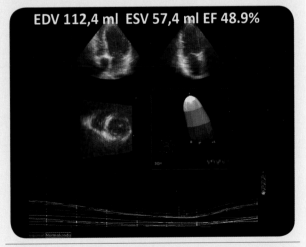

Video 2.6. 3D quantification of left ventricular function (EF 48.9%)

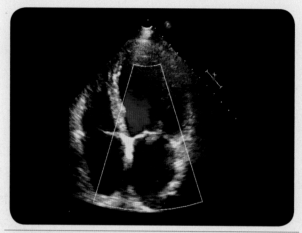

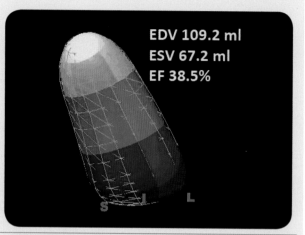

EDV 109.2 ml
ESV 67.2 ml
EF 38.5%

Video 2.7. 2D color apical four-chamber view showed mild mitral regurgitation after EF improvement

Video 2.8. 3D full-volume quantification of 3D-ejection fraction, showed a 10% asymptomatic decrease in EF

Figures

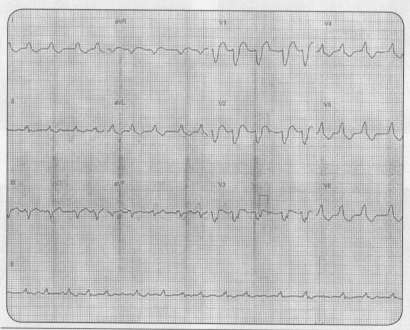

Figure 2.1. 12-lead ECG recording on admission. Rapid atrial fibrillation with left bundle branch block

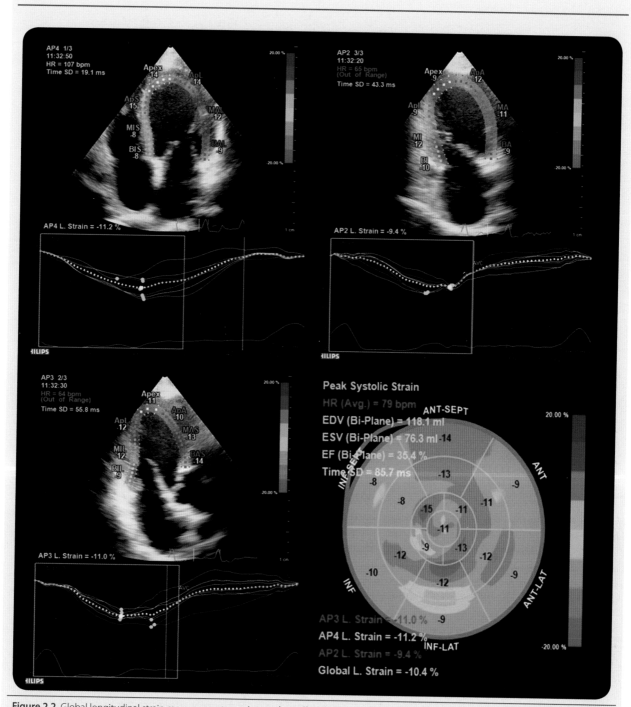

Figure 2.2. Global longitudinal strain measurement remains at a low value despite improvements in ejection fraction

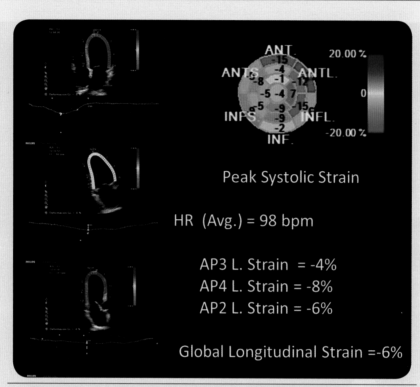

Figure 2.3. Follow-up global longitudinal strain remains above -12%

2.2. Discussion

Chemotherapy can promote a variety of toxicities; among the most severe are those involving the cardiovascular system. Due to the aging and increasingly complex nature of our patients, cardiac risk stratification before establishment of a cancer treatment is mandatory in order to try to reduce cardiovascular side effects and to deliver the treatment in a more patient-centered fashion early.

Patients over the age of 75 or with extensive cardiovascular co-morbidities have an increased risk of developing heart failure if exposed to potentially cardiotoxic drugs. A detailed risk algorithm taking into account treatment toxicities and pre-existing cardiovascular conditions would be helpful in managing these populations.

Anthracyclines are the prototype drugs of type I chemotherapy-induced cardiotoxicity. Traditionally, a distinction has been made between acute (< 1 month), subacute and a chronic (> 1 year) anthracyline-induced cardiotoxicity. The acute and subacute forms develop at the time or within the first months of administration of anthracyclines and resemble an acute myocarditis. Chronic cardiotoxicity was considered to be irreversible and refractory to standard heart failure therapy. However, a combined strategy of close surveillance and early institution of targeted therapy allows for recovery of ejection fraction in most patients. The treatment of heart failure in the setting of cardiotoxicity should follow the same rules established for any other heart failure scenarios.

In this case a complete recovery of left ventricular function was not achieved probably because of previous subclinical baseline damage due to pre-existent diabetes and dyslipidemia. Even in the absence of a baseline quantification of deformation parameters, after left ventricular ejection fraction (LVEF) partially recovered, global longitudinal strain (GLS) remained above -12%. LVEF has been established as the routine prognostic parameter of LV global dysfunction. However, recently there is strong evidence supporting the superior prognostic value of GLS over standard LVEF, for major adverse cardiac events. GLS measured by 2D-speckle has been demonstrated in clinical populations to improve cardiac risk stratification. A GLS ≥ -12% is equivalent to a severely depressed LVEF (Stanton T, Leano R and Marwick TH. Prediction of all-cause mortality from global longitudinal speckle strain: comparison with ejection fraction and wall motion scoring. *Circ Cardiovasc Imaging.* 2009 Sep; 2(5): 356-364). Guidelines incorporating measures of LV function may need to be revised in order to incorporate global longitudinal strain in light of these findings.

Atrial fibrillation, a common finding in the elderly, can be exacerbated by anticancer treatments and complicate overall course.

Finally, the use of cardio-protective agents, like statins, beta-blockers, or ACEI, can prevent chemotherapy-related cardiotoxicity, reducing cardiac-related mortality and morbidity. In this case the use of statins or ACEI in the pre-chemotherapy phase could have reduced cardiovascular side effects.

2.3. Conclusions

In cancers with high probability of long-term survival, it is very important to consider cardiovascular risks. Pre-existing medical conditions modify the risk of cardiotoxicity in cancer patients. There is a need for cooperation between cardiologists and onco-hematologists to move toward a protective chemoprevention approach, in order to reduce cardiotoxicity.

Case 03

Cardiogenic Shock after Chemotherapy Treatment

Silvia Valbuena López
Oscar González Fernández

Cardiology Department. La Paz University Hospital. IdiPAz Research Institute. Madrid. Spain

3.1. Case Presentation

A previously healthy 38-year-old male was diagnosed with an infiltrative colorectal adenocarcinoma with four metastatic liver lesions. After careful evaluation by the Oncology and General Surgery team, neoadyuvant therapy followed by surgical removal of the tumor with curative intent was planned. Treatment with 5-fluorouracil (5-FU) and oxaliplatin was started, initially with uneventful course.

However, 24 hours after the first drug infusion, the patient presented with retrosternal oppressive chest pain of high intensity, which did not change with movements or breathing and was not accompanied by fever. He was initially admitted to the cardiology ward, but his condition worsened rapidly, presenting with an acute pulmonary edema and evidence of a severe left ventricular dysfunction in an emergency echocardiography **(Video 3.1, Video 3.2, Video 3.3, Video 3.4, Video 3.5, and Video 3.6).**

Physical exam revealed blood pressure 70/50 mmHg, heart rate 120 bpm with a third sound, and bilateral fine crackles. Highest Troponin I value was 4 ng/mL (normal range < 0.02), and ECG showed sinus tachycardia with diffuse ST elevation. He was transferred to the Coronary Unit where he required orotracheal intubation and mechanical ventilation, inotropic support, and placement of an intra-aortic balloon pump. He also suffered multiple episodes of supraventricular and ventricular tachycardia, and three episodes of ventricular fibrillation.

After 72 hours hemodynamic stability was achieved and support measures could be progressively withdrawn. Clinical course was positive and eventually low dose ACEI and beta-blockers could be started. Coronary disease was excluded with a multidetector cardiac computed tomography and a cardiac magnetic resonance was performed in order to reassess LVEF and to obtain etiologic information about the event. It showed a normal LVEF, with slight lateral and apical hypokinesis **(Video 3.7).** Triple inversion-recovery T2-weighted images were consistent with edema and inflammation in the lateral wall **(Figure 3.1),** and intramyocardial late gadolinium hyperenhacement was observed in the same location. These findings were consistent with acute myocarditis; 15 days after his admission, the patient was finally discharged with the diagnosis of toxic myocarditis due to cardiotoxic drugs, under treatment with ACEI and beta-blockers.

Due to the life-threatening cardiac complications that he had suffered, the patient was directly referred for surgery, achieving the total removal of the colorectal tumor and the liver metastasis. However, in a control computed tomography performed three months after surgery, new focal liver lesions had appeared, and therapy with cetuximab and irinotecan was started, with poor response and hepatic and retroperitoneal progression of the disease. A new scheme with oxaliplatin, bevacizumab, and ralitrexed was proposed. Given the previous cardiotoxicity, the patient was admitted for careful cardiac monitoring of the first infusion, with excellent tolerance. The disease was stabilized for some months, but the patient finally died after 15 months.

Videos

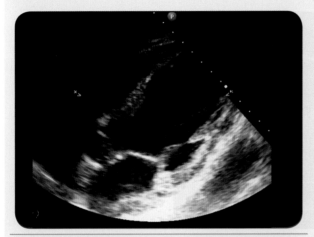

Video 3.1. Parasternal long-axis showing severely impaired LVEF

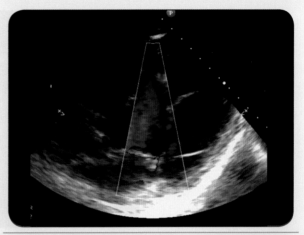

Video 3.2. Parasternal long-axis color-Doppler image shows mild mitral regurgitation

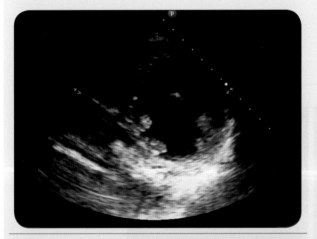

Video 3.3. Parasternal short-axis view showing severely impaired LVEF

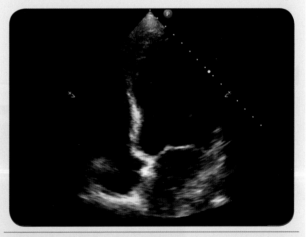

Video 3.4. Apical four-chamber view showing a severe global hypokinesis

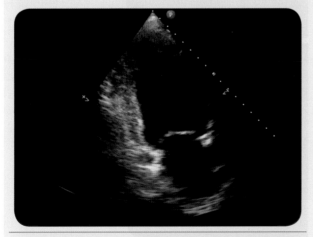

Video 3.5. Apical two-chamber view. Normal mitral valve with thin leaflets, and with no closure restriction can be observed

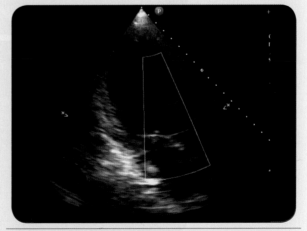

Video 3.6. Apical three-chamber view color-Doppler. Despite the severe impairment of LVEF, no coaptation defect exists, with only mild mitral regurgitation

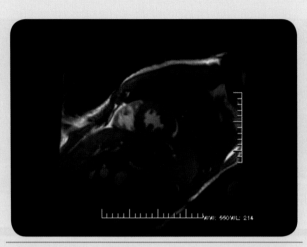

Video 3.7. Short-axis cine-MRI sequence that confirms a striking improvement in LV function, with almost normal global contractility

Figures

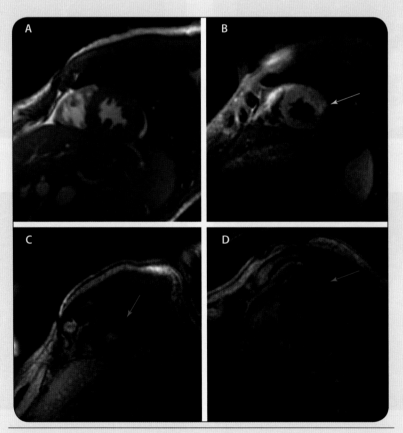

Figure 3.1. Short-axis cine-MRI images. **A:** still image from cine mode; **B:** myocardial edema *(yellow arrow)* in the STIR view. **C** and **D:** post-contrast T1 short-axis and four-chamber views, showing intramyocardial late gadolinium enhancement in the lateral wall of LV *(red arrow)*

3.2. Discussion

This case illustrates an acute manifestation of drug-induced cardiotoxicity. Although it is not as common as chronic cardiotoxicity, its relatively high mortality and devastating effects should be kept in mind whenever patients receive potentially cardiotoxic drugs. 5-FU is an active antimetabolite used for the treatment of a variety of gastrointestinal, pancreatic, breast, bladder, and prostatic cancer, all of which have scarce effective alternative therapeutic regimens. The incidence of cardiotoxicity varies between 0.55% and 8% in different series, and comprises a wide spectrum of clinical manifestations, such as myocardial ischemia (vasospasm mediated or secondary to coronary thrombosis), arrhythmias, heart failure, or myopericarditis. Most events develop within the first cycle of chemotherapy, as in our case. Therefore, any symptoms that appear hours or days after the infusion of 5-FU should raise the suspicion of a cardiac event, and prompt assessment of LV function or myocardial ischemia. Whenever any abnormalities are found, careful monitoring is recommended, as quick worsening and development of cardiogenic shock can occur within hours.

Although the use of oxaliplatin does not definitively involve a higher risk of cardiotoxicity, it predisposes to arrhythmias, and in combination with 5-FU it could increase cardiac adverse events.

In our case, although the patient did not have any risk factors or previous structural heart disease, he developed cardiogenic shock requiring advanced support measures. MRI provided useful data regarding the etiology of the LV dysfunction, suggesting toxic acute myocarditis. Similar presentations have been previously reported related to the use of 5-FU, with marked improvement after cessation of the drug. Due to the advanced oncologic disease of this patient, chemotherapy was considered to be essential, and careful consideration of the risk/benefit ratio should have been taken place before withdrawal of such an important drug. As the risk of recurrence of CT when patients are re-challenged with 5-FU is known to be high, ralitrexed seemed to be a reasonable substitute of 5-FU with a better risk profile. However, as the disease progressed, oxaliplatin was restarted without developing further cardiac complications.

3.3. Conclusions

Acute cardiotoxicity has been related to a variety of cancer drugs through different mechanisms. Symptoms or signs of heart failure or myocardial ischemia after receiving potentially cardiotoxic drugs must trigger a rapid response and cardiac evaluation, as these events often have significant mortality and morbidity.

Case 04

Acute Pericarditis during Radiation Therapy

Oscar González Fernández
Silvia Valbuena López

Cardiology Department. La Paz University Hospital. IdiPAz Research Institute. Madrid. Spain

4.1. Case Presentation

A 58-year-old white woman with breast cancer was admitted to the hospital because of chest pain and fever in January 2014. The patient had a previous history of deficit of activated protein C with past axillary and subclavian vein thrombosis treated with acenocumarol, which was finally suspended due to an intracranial hemorrhage.

In July 2013, she was diagnosed with a left breast carcinoma. The mammography performed at that time revealed an architectural distortion of the left breast and a non-calcified small cyst; the biopsy was compatible with a grade 2 invasive ductal carcinoma, positive for human epidermal growth factor receptor 2 (HER2/neu) as well as estrogen and progesterone receptors, with 10% Ki67 expression. No further tissue invasion was detected. She underwent neo-adjuvant therapy with cyclophosphamide and epirubicin; followed by conservative tumorectomy and combined adjuvant therapy with an aromatase inhibitor (letrozole 2.5 mg daily), trastuzumab, as well as radiotherapy (50Gy; 2Gy/day).

The patient was doing well until January 2014, when she developed fever and chest pain while ongoing radiotherapy cycles. The chest pain was sharp and pleuritic, improving by sitting up and leaning forward. On examination blood pressure was 115/68 mmHg, heart rate was 70 bpm, temperature was 36.5 °C, and oxygen saturation was 98% while she was breathing ambient air. Carotid pulse and jugular veins were normal. Heart sounds were rhythmic and a pericardial rub was heard. Lungs were clear.

An electrocardiogram revealed sinus rhythm at a rate of 92 bpm and diffuse concave up ST elevation with reciprocal ST depression in lead aVR **(Figure 4.1)**. A chest X-ray was normal. Blood test showed hematocrit of 42.4%, white-cell count of 15,000/μL with an elevated percentage of band forms (89%), platelet count of 177,000/μL. Sodium, potassium, chloride, glucose, serial troponin, creatinine, and C-reactive protein were normal. No pericardial effusion and preserved systolic function with normal aortic and mitral valves were shown in the emergency echocardiography **(Video 4.1, Video 4.2, Video 4.3, Video 4.4, and Video 4.5)**.

With the diagnose of acute pericarditis, the patient was treated for two weeks with non-steroidal anti-inflammatory drugs (ibuprofen 600 mg, three times daily) with pain relief after the first dose. No more fever spikes were registered after treatment establishment. In a follow-up visit two weeks after discharge, she remained asymptomatic, no pericardial rub was documented on physical exam and the ECG was compatible with sinus rhythm at a rate of 68 beats per minute with T-wave inversion in leads V1- V3. Echocardiogram revealed no pericardial effusion and preserved systolic ejection fraction **(Video 4.6)**. Radiotherapy was completed one week after the event.

Two months later, the patient developed an episode of paroxysmal atrial fibrillation, so anticoagulation with dabigatran and rate control strategies with bisoprolol were started. No further pericarditis episodes occurred. Twelve months later the patient undergoes regular follow-up without recurrences.

Videos

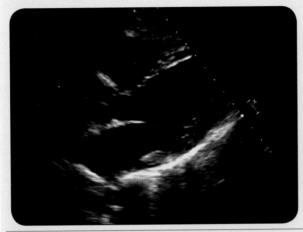

Video 4.1. Parasternal long-axis view showing preserved left ventricular function with normal mitral and aortic valves

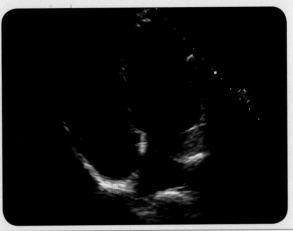

Video 4.2. Apical four-chamber view showing preserved left ventricular function with normal mitral and aortic valves and no pericardial effusion

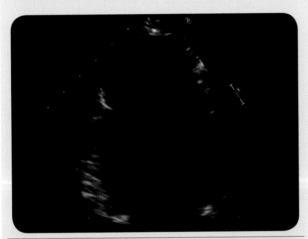

Video 4.3. Apical two-chamber view showing preserved left ventricular function with normal mitral valve and no pericardial effusion

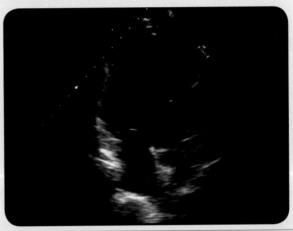

Video 4.4. Apical three-chamber view showing preserved left ventricular function with normal mitral and aortic valves and no pericardial effusion

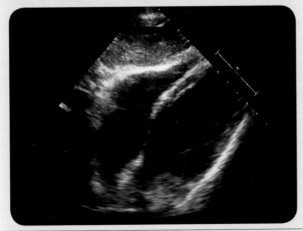

Video 4.5. Subcostal four-chamber view showing no pericardial effusion and preserved left ventricular systolic function

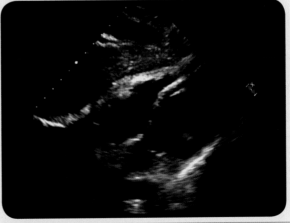

Video 4.6. Subcostal four-chamber view after two weeks reveals no pericardial effusion

Figures

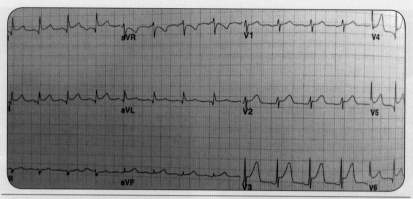

Figure 4.1. Sinus rhythm at a rate of 92 bpm and diffuse concave up ST elevation with reciprocal ST depression in lead aVR

4.2. Discussion

This clinical case illustrates the development of acute pericarditis after radiation therapy. Breast cancer treatment has been related to cardiotoxic effects. Every heart structure is susceptible to radiation effects, pericardial disease being the most common cardiac complication. Radiation delivered at therapeutic doses predisposes to the formation of deposits of collagen and fibrin in the pericardium. Major determinants of cardiotoxicity include total radiation dose, dose per session, exposed heart volume and use of concomitant chemotherapy. Doses higher than 35-40 Gy, or fractionated doses more than 2 Gy are considered to be risk factors for radiation-induced pericardial disease. Pericardial disease may manifest acutely during radiation therapy as pericarditis, or years later as constrictive pericarditis, effusive-constrictive pericarditis, pericardial effusion, or pericardial tamponade.

In the last decade, the incidence of pericarditis has significantly decreased due to the introduction of changes in method for the delivery of radiation therapy. About 20% of patients with acute pericarditis finally develop constrictive or chronic pericarditis over a period of five to 10 years after treatment completion. The risk for developing chronic pericarditis is substantially greater if there was previous pericardial effusion. Acute pericarditis should be treated with non-steroidal anti-inflammatory drugs such as ibuprofen, indomethacin, or aspirin.

European guidelines recommend ibuprofen as the reference drug. If the patient develops cardiac tamponade pericardiocentesis should be performed.

In our case, the patient developed acute pericarditis during radiation therapy. The radiation dose administered was 50 Gy, slightly higher than total recommended dose to avoid complications. The patient remained stable, without development of pericardial effusion and excellent clinical response to non-steroidal anti-inflammatory drugs. Stopping or modifying radiation therapy after an episode of acute pericarditis should be considered depending on the risk/benefit ratio. In our case the patient completed every radiation therapy session, ceasing treatment one week after the event.

4.3. Conclusions

Patients undergoing chemotherapy and radiation therapy may develop cardiotoxicity and should be closely monitored. Current radiation therapy regimens have substantially decreased the risk of cardiotoxicity. Radiation-induced cardiac damage can involve all structures of the heart, pericardial disease being the most common cardiac complication. Radiation-induced pericarditis should be treated with non-steroidal anti-inflammatory drugs, and according to the risk/benefit ratio radiotherapy can be modified.

Case 05

Valvulopathy Induced by Radiotherapy

Alberto Cecconi
Pedro Martínez Losas

Cardiology Department. San Carlos University Hospital. Madrid. Spain

5.1. Case Presentation

A 34-year-old woman in the 32.nd week of gestation presented to the emergency department with a 10-day story of progressive shortness of breath. She was diagnosed 13 years before with a Hodgkin's lymphoma and treated with chemotherapy (doxorubicin, bleomycin, vinblastine, darcarbacine, and prednisolone) and with mediastinal radiotherapy (40 Gy), achieving complete remission. She denied any history of rheumatic fever. Since of week 20 pregnancy, she was receiving treatment with labetalol for gestational hypertension.

On arrival, she was tachycardic and tachypneic with a blood pressure of 192/120 mmHg and an oxygen saturation of 89% on room air. Widespread inspiratory lung crackles and a holosystolic murmur best heard at the cardiac apex radiating to the axilla was present. A symmetric pitting edema was observed in both legs. ECG revealed a sinus tachycardia **(Figure 5.1)** and chest X-ray confirmed signs of pulmonary edema. Complete blood count, renal function, coagulation times, and liver function tests were normal. Troponin I and NTproBNP were 0.09 ng/mL (normal values < 0.05 ng/mL) and 2,100 (normal values < 450 pg/mL), respectively. A mild proteinuria of 250 mg/day was detected. Echocardiography revealed a mitral valve thickening with retraction and reduced motion of the posterior leaflet, resulting in a coaptation defect and a jet of severe mitral regurgitation. A mild enlargement of the left atrium was seen, while dimensions and motility of the left ventricle were normal **(Video 5.1, Video 5.2, and Video 5.3).** The pattern of disease of the mitral valve was suggestive of damage due to previous radiotherapy.

A diagnosis of acute heart failure caused by valvular dysfunction due to radiotherapy with severe mitral regurgitation worsened by gestational hypertension was made, and treatment with intravenous diuretic, nitrates, labetalol, and non-invasive ventilation was commenced. Given the lack of response to medical therapy and worsening of respiratory failure, the patient underwent emergency cesarean surgery. Subsequently, clinical course of heart failure was satisfactory and her recovery was uneventful. Three months after discharge, the patient was asymptomatic and mitral regurgitation was moderate on echocardiography.

Videos

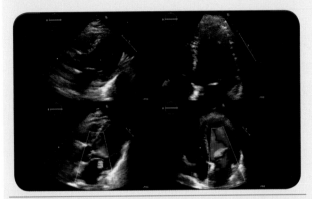

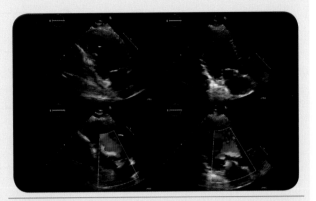

Video 5.1. TTE evaluation. Parasternal *(left)* and four-chamber *(right)* views in 2D *(upper line)* and color *(lower line)* modes showing retraction and reduced motion of the posterior leaflet and severe mitral regurgitation

Video 5.2. TTE evaluation. Two-chamber *(left)* and three-chamber *(right)* views in 2D *(upper line)* and color *(lower line)* modes showing retraction and reduced motion of the posterior leaflet and severe mitral regurgitation

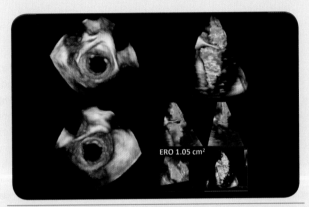

Video 5.3. Transesophageal-3D evaluation of the mitral valve. Views from auricular *(left and up)* and ventricular *(left and down)* sides of the valve showing retraction of the posterior leaflet and an abnormal widening of the closure line that causes a wide coaptation defect. 3D-color mode *(upper right)* reveals severe mitral regurgitation. MPR images from 3D-color Doppler *(lower right)* can be used for ERO measurement by means of vena contracta planimetry. The result (1.05 cm²) is consistent with severe mitral regurgitation

Figures

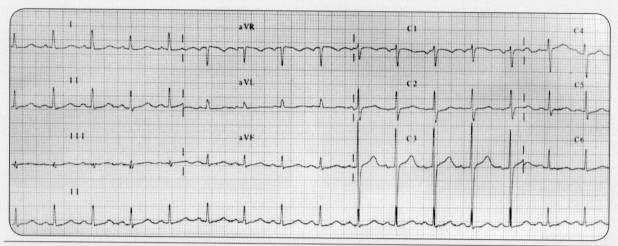

Figure 5.1. ECG on ER admission. Sinus tachycardia is observed

5.2. Discussion

This case illustrates a common cardiac complication of thoracic irradiation. Although radiotherapy has led to a significant improvement in the treatment of thoracic cancers, the benefits are partially counterbalanced by long-term cardiac alterations. Indeed, cardiovascular disease is the most common non-malignant cause of death among patients with Hodgkin's lymphoma and breast cancer treated with radiotherapy.

Thoracic radiotherapy can affect all of the heart structures. Typically, pericarditis might be the acute manifestation, whereas chronic pericardial disease, valvular abnormalities, systolic and diastolic dysfunction, coronary artery disease, and conduction disturbances might appear over decades after exposure. The incidence of valvular dysfunction increases during the second decade after mediastinal radiotherapy for Hodgkin's Lymphoma. Mitral and aortic valves are affected more than right-sided valves, probably due to the higher pressure of left-sided chambers. Leaflet retraction appears to be the early valvular change, while thickening, calcification, and stenosis develop over decades. If a surgical intervention is necessary, valve replacement seems to be the best choice, since durability of valve repair is limited.

Several risk factors for radiation-associated heart damage have been recognized, including: dose > 30-35 Gy, dose per fraction > 2 Gy, younger age at exposure, large volume of irradiated heart, longer time since exposure, and use of chemotherapeutic drugs such as anthracyclines and trastuzumab.

Long-term cardiac follow-up is mandatory in patients who received thoracic radiotherapy in order to enable early detection of cardiac complications. In asymptomatic patients, cardiac screening should commence five years post exposure. In addition, any woman who has received thoracic radiation should be assessed by a cardiologist in case of pregnancy.

5.3. Conclusions

Thoracic irradiation has a high incidence of long-term cardiac complications. Clinicians should consider patients treated with thoracic radiotherapy as high-risk for cardiac events. Echocardiography is a reliable technique for screening cardiac adverse effects in asymptomatic patients.

Case 06

Chest Pain in a Radiotherapy Patient

Pedro Martínez Losas
Carmen Olmos Blanco

Cardiology Department. San Carlos University Hospital. Madrid. Spain

6.1. Case Presentation

A 59-year-old woman with previous history of hypertension and dyslipidemia was treated for breast cancer stage T2N1M0 (hormone receptor negative and HER-2 positive) with CEF, paclitaxel, and trastuzumab, as well as radiotherapy and surgery (bilateral mastectomy, ipsilateral axillary lymphadenectomy, and breast reconstruction) achieving good results and complete remission of the disease. The patient continued maintenance therapy with trastuzumab and control CT scan revealed no tumor recurrence. However, three months after treatment, the patient developed neuropathy, severe asthenia, breathlessness on exercise, and episodes of chest pain.

A cardiologic evaluation was started. Echocardiography showed normal LVEF and GLS -15% **(Video 6.1, Video 6.2, and Video 6.3)**. The GLS value was lower than expected and medical treatment with beta-blocker and ACEI was started. Chest pain complaints were studied with an exercise test, with negative results but low functional status (four minutes of exercise, 5 METS). The exercise test was inconclusive because the peak heart rate achieved was lower than 85% of the maximum expected. This is the reason why a CT scan was ordered and showed no coronary disease **(Figure 6.4)**. One year later, the patient did not have other cardiovascular symptoms and follow-up TTE showed normalization of the GLS values.

Videos

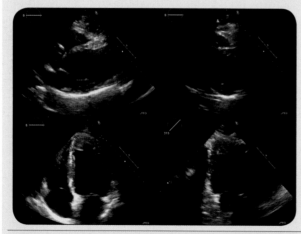

Video 6.1. Transthoracic echo reveals normal left ventricular function and normal valvular anatomy

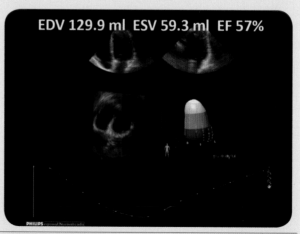

Video 6.2. 3D evaluation of left ventricular function. Global and regional contractility were normal

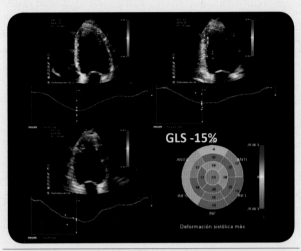

Video 6.3. Deformation study showed a normal GLS

Figures

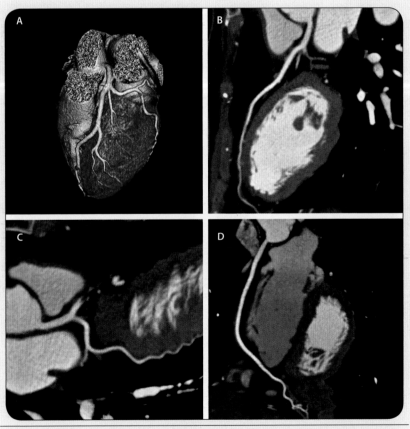

Figure 6.1. Cardiac CT for coronary evaluation. **A:** volume render of the heart. Left anterior descending **(B)**, circumflex **(C)** and right **(D)** coronary arteries were free of disease

6.2. Discussion

Treatment of patients with cancer has improved over recent decades thanks to a combination of early diagnosis and better treatment. The result is a global increase in survival rates, but also in the development of cardiac comorbidities during follow-up. Cardiac evaluation before chemotherapy and during follow-up is critical to unveil cardiovascular problems and to start cardiac treatment before symptoms develop. This strategy is linked to a better prognosis in the long-term.

This case study represents a good example of these clinical problems. A patient operated for breast cancer, who received chemotherapy and radiotherapy complained of dyspnea, asthenia, and episodes of chest pain. Symptoms can be caused by tumor recurrence, undesired effects of the treatment or by the development of a new cardiac disease.

The cardiologist should be aware of possible cardiovascular effects of cancer therapy. The most frequent problem is the development of ventricular dysfunction produced by anthracyclines, cyclophosphamide, or trastuzumab. However, there could also be undesired vascular effects of 5-fluorouracil (vasospasm) or vascular damage due to radiotherapy. Radiotherapy has also been linked to pericarditis (the most frequent complication), heart disease, valvular heart disease, and myocardiopathy. Risk is related to the amount of radiation received and the area to which it is delivered. Vascular damage due to radiotherapy is usually seen in the long-term, 5-10 years after therapy. However the coexistence of other vascular risk factors (like hypertension) can cause coronary disease to develop faster.

Every patient should be carefully evaluated at baseline by taking a full medical history and detailed physical examination to assess their base cardiovascular risk. A chest X-ray, an ECG, and an echocardiography are also recommended. This initial examination, along with disease course, treatment and appearance of symptoms, allows us to determine the correct type of follow-up. Basic guidelines for cardiac evaluation are the same as for non-oncologic patients with extreme care paid to a need to change oncologic therapy. In our case, there was a need to rule out coronary disease and the patient was a evaluated by stress testing and coronary CT scan.

6.3. Conclusions

The increase in survival rates of cancer patients is linked to the increase in cardiovascular problems that can be caused by the disease, the treatment or development of a new cardiac condition. This is the cause of the development of a new concept, cardio-oncology, where the intervention of the cardiologist in the decision-making process is increasing.

The presence of symptoms that suggest a cardiovascular origin during the course of the illness should be a reason for assessment.

Case 07

Subclinical Left Ventricular Dysfunction after Chemotheraphy Treatment

Juan Caro Codón
Sandra Rosillo Rodríguez

Cardiology Department. La Paz University Hospital. IdiPAz Research Institute. Madrid. Spain

7.1. Case Presentation

A 31-year-old man, without past medical history, was diagnosed with acute promyelocytic leukemia with high-risk features and was referred to our hospital for a complete evaluation by the hematology department. Genetic tests confirmed the presence of t(15:17) and lp53 mutations, and a decision was made to initiate treatment with all-trans retinoic acid and idarubicin (21 mg). The patient subsequently received two cycles of consolidation chemotherapy with idarubicin (8.6 mg), cytarabine (1,700 mg), and mitoxantrone (17 mg), and presented two episodes of febrile neutropenia that resolved after treatment with broad-spectrum antibiotics.

Before the administration of chemotherapy, transthoracic echocardiography **(Figure 7.1, Figure 7.2, and Video 7.1)** showed normal biventricular systolic function (LVEF 58%), absence of regional wall-motion abnormalities, and global longitudinal strain (GLS) within normal limits (GLS -18%). After treatment, initial follow-up transthoracic echocardiographies showed normal systolic function and deformation parameters, but a subsequent study performed seven months after the initiation of oncologic treatment, while the patient was free of cardiac symptoms, revealed a marked decline in GLS to -13 **(Figure 7.3),** with a LVEF in the low range of normality (53%).

An active surveillance strategy was adopted. The patient was seen in an outpatient setting during the following three weeks. He gradually developed dyspnea on moderate exertion, and echocardiography confirmed abnormal longitudinal strain (GLS -12%) with normal ejection fraction **(Figure 7.4, Video 7.2, and Video 7.3).** Beta-blocker treatment was started, with good tolerance. Over the following months, cardiac symptoms progressively resolved and subsequent echocardiography **(Figure 7.5 and Video 7.4)** confirmed normal values of LVEF (62%) and myocardial deformation parameters (GLS -18%).

Videos

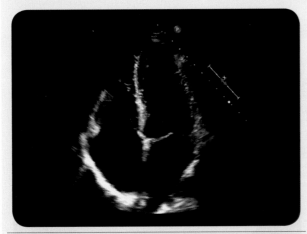

Video 7.1. Apical four-chamber view showed preserved LVEF without regional wall motion abnormalities

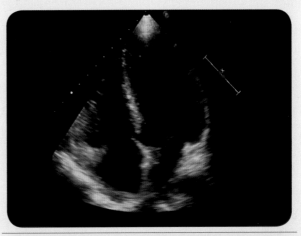

Video 7.2. Despite the decline in GLS, apical four-chamber view shows normal contractility

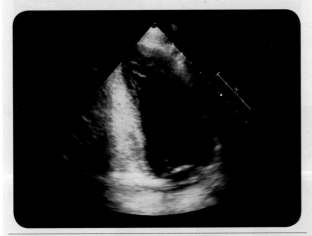

Video 7.3. Apical two-chamber also showed normal systolic function without evident wall motion abnormalities

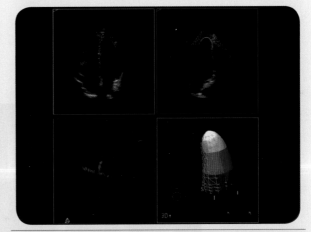

Video 7.4. Left ventricular 3D analysis confirmed normal LV contractility after normalization of global longitudinal strain

Figures

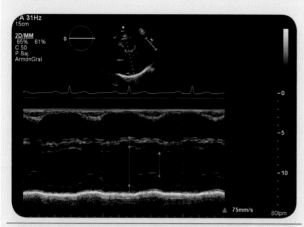

Figure 7.1. M-mode echocardiography of the left ventricle showing normal left ventricular ejection fraction

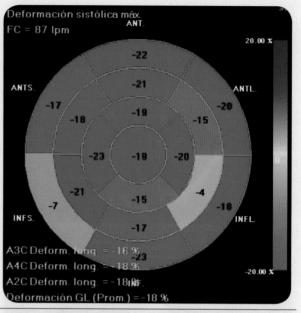

Figure 7.2. Bull's eye view analysis of global longitudinal strain showed values within normal limits

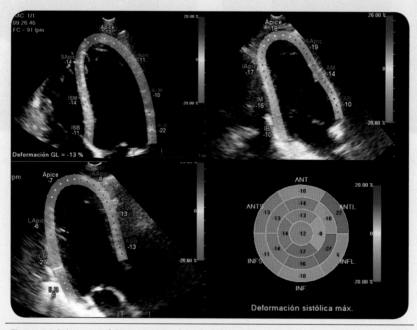

Figure 7.3 Subsequent follow-up showed marked decline in GLS

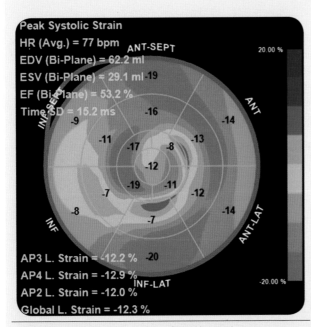

Figure 7.4. Low GLS values were confirmed by serial echocardiography during active cardiac monitoring

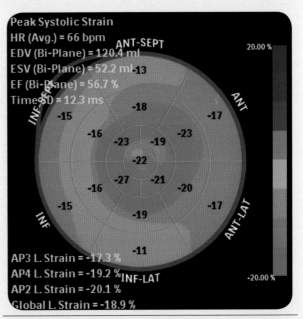

Figure 7.5. Bull's eye view analysis of GLS after five months of beta-blocker therapy confirmed normal strain values

7.2. Discussion

In recent years, the multidisciplinary approach of cancer patients has led to better knowledge of cardiac effects associated with chemotherapy, as well as their clinical implications. Strategies for the early diagnosis and management of cardiac toxicity have also been developed.

A significant percentage of patients treated with anthra-cyclines will develop myocardial damage that may lead to major cardiovascular events and cardiac failure-related hospitalizations, becoming one of the most important causes of morbidity in this population.

Although anthracycline-related cardiac toxicity was previously considered to be irreversible, early detection and prompt treatment with ACEIs and beta-blockers may prevent adverse left ventricular remodeling and progression to heart failure symptoms.

Therefore, one of the key points in the management of cancer therapeutics-related cardiac dysfunction is the development of specific methods that may improve detection of sub-clinical cardiac damage.

LVEF is the most commonly used parameter to measure systolic function and is clearly related to long-term prognosis, both in the general population and in specific sub-settings like oncologic patients.

Nevertheless, accurate calculation of LVEF has several limitations including geometric assumptions, lack of consideration of subtle wall-motion abnormalities and inherent intra- and inter-observer variability. 3D-Echo overcomes the limitations of 2D-Echo, but even the best LVEF method still does not detect myocardial damage at an early stage.

On the other side, there is a growing body of evidence regarding several advanced echocardiographic techniques that may improve early detection of subclinical LV dysfunction. Systolic deformation indices are becoming a useful tool in the management of these patients, because they may predict the development of clinical events during follow-up.

In our patient, routine echocardiographic follow-up showed a significant decrease in global longitudinal strain, which is the optimal parameter of deformation for early detection of sub-clinical left ventricular dysfunction. Changes in GLS precede deterioration of LVEF and and favor prompt initiation of cardiac treatment.

Animal and human research has focused on the hypothesis that prophylactic pharmacologic intervention in all patients receiving chemotherapy may prevent left ventricular dysfunction and heart failure. Nevertheless, the optimal approach seems to be a strategy of early detection and treatment of myocardial disease, avoiding use of unnecessary drugs (and their adverse effects) in patients without cardiac damage.

7.3. Conclusions

This case illustrates the usefulness of GLS as a technique that may improve screening of chemotherapy-related cardiac toxicity and further guide the decision to initiate treatment aimed at preventing adverse cardiac remodeling, even before a decrease in LVEF occurs or heart failure symptoms appear.

Case 08

Chemotherapy and Chest Radiation as Risk Factor for Cardiotoxicity: How to Manage this High Risk Population

Silvia Valbuena López
Oscar González Fernández

Cardiology Department. La Paz University Hospital. IdiPAz Research Institute. Madrid. Spain

8.1. Case Presentation

A 48-year-old female, with a previous history of hypertension and mild lupus nephropathy was diagnosed with a locally advanced left breast cancer in 2001. At the time of diagnosis she was treated with enalapril and diltiazem. She underwent conservative surgery, where six axillar lymphnodes were found to be affected. The immuno-histologic analysis of tumoral tissue was negative for hormonal receptors and HER2+. Adjuvant therapy with epirubicin-cyclophosphamide and paclitaxel, followed by radiotherapy (total delivery dose of 45 Gy in 2 Gy daily fraction and extra boost of 10 Gy) was scheduled.

She had an uneventful course until January 2010, when she presented with skin lesions in her left breast and a marked elevation of Ca19.9. Breast magnetic resonance showed extensive relapse of the tumor in her left breast, with satellite nodes affecting all four quadrants and bilateral metastatic adenopathies; cytology of the skin lesions confirmed the presence of cancerous HER2+ cells. An echocardiography was performed prior to a new chemotherapy regimen, showed a normal-sized left ventricle with preserved ejection fraction (LVEF) **(Video 8.1, Video 8.2, and Video 8.3).** However, the mitral valve was slightly calcified with a grade II/IV mitral regurgitation **(Video 8.4).** Chemotherapy with eight cycles of docetaxel plus traztuzumab was administered, followed by left mastectomy and resection of bilateral lymph nodes. After surgery, trastuzumab treatment was restarted in association with carboplatin.

After five months, chemotherapy was switched because of cutaneous and right breast relapse of the tumor. Liposomal doxorubicin and lapatinib were then started. But nine months afterwards, skin disease progressed and treatment was switched to a gemcitabin/paclitaxel/traztuzumab/lapatinib scheme. Disease stabilization was achieved for two years. The patient remained asymptomatic, with no routine follow-up echo evaluation until October 2013, when slightly dilated left ventricle with global hypokinesis and moderate left ventricular dysfunction (LVEF 40%; **Video 8.5, Video 8.6, Video 8.7, and Video 8.8),** as well as severely calcified mitral valve with severe MR **(Video 8.9, Video 8.10 and Video 8.11)** were detected. The right ventricle was normal-sized but ejection fraction was moderately depressed.

Following these findings trastuzumab was discontinued and the patient was referred for cardiology consultation. Diltiazem was stopped, enalapril doses were optimized and bisoprolol therapy was started. After two months a new echocardiography was performed, showing a significant improvement in LVEF **(Video 8.12, Video 8.13, and Video 8.14)** and persistent severe mitral regurgitation **(Video 8.15, Vídeo 8.16 and Figure 8.1).** After discussion of the cardio-oncology team, traztuzumab was restarted, due to the improvement in LVEF and the poor prognosis of her oncologic disease. Optimization of cardioprotective drugs and close cardiac monitoring was performed, with no further significant changes in echocardiographic findings.

Videos

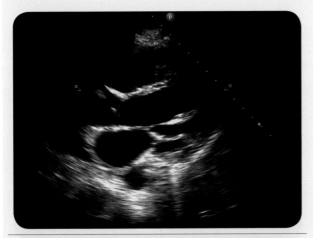

Video 8.1. Parasternal long-axis view showing a normal-sized left ventricle with no regional contraction abnormalities

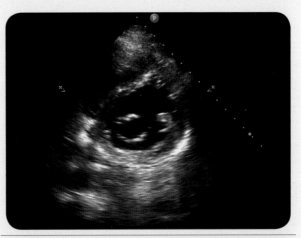

Video 8.2. Parasternal short-axis view, at the level of the mitral valve, whose leaflets are slightly thickened and calcified

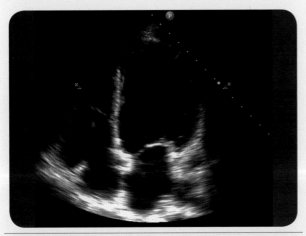

Video 8.3. Apical four-chamber view, where a normal LVEF can be observed (LVEF with Simpson biplane method 59%)

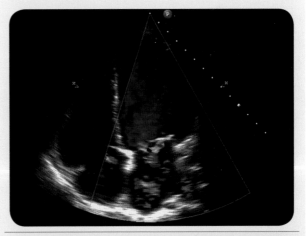

Video 8.4. Color-Doppler apical four-chamber view. A grade II/IV mitral regurgitation is present, secondary to mitral valve thickening

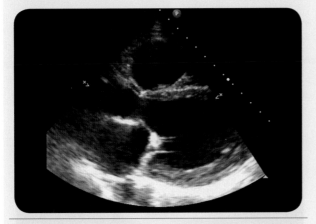

Video 8.5. Parasternal long-axis view. Slightly dilated LV with global hypokinesis and severe calcification of both leaflets of the mitral valve can be observed

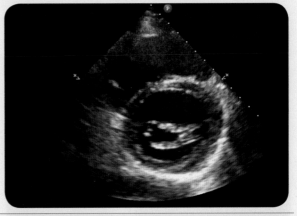

Video 8.6. Parasternal short-axis view, which shows severe thickening and calcification of both leaflets of the mitral valve, without opening restriction

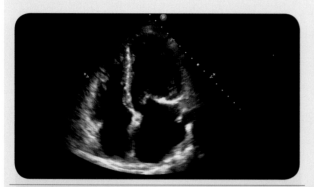

Video 8.7. Apical four-chamber view. Global hypokinesis, with moderately depressed left ventricle function is present, with a LVEF calculated with the Simpson biplane method of 40%. Right ventricle is also slightly hypokinetic, and left atrium is moderately enlarged. Mitral valve involvement is also appreciated in these views, mainly affecting the posterior leaflet

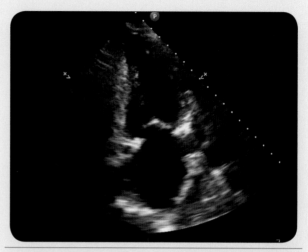

Video 8.8. Apical two-chamber view. See Video 8.7

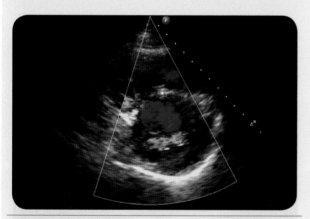

Video 8.9. Color-Doppler parasternal short-axis view showing a pansystolic regurgitation jet along the whole coaptation line of both mitral leaflets

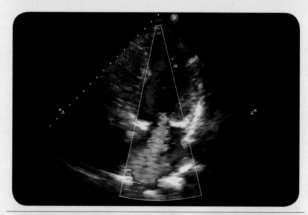

Video 8.10. Color-Doppler four-chamber apical view, where a severe mitral regurgitation can be observed. The regurgitating jet is pansystolic, eccentric, aimed towards the posterior wall of the left atrium, and enters the right inferior pulmonary vein, where systolic flow is reversed

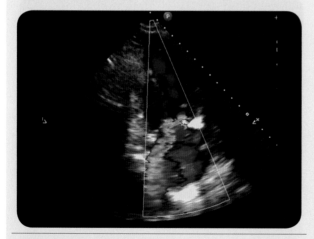

Video 8.11. Color-Doppler two-chamber apical view. See Video 8.10

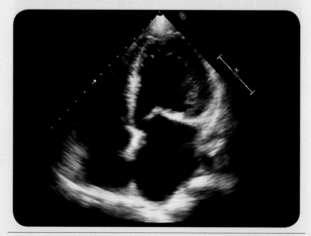

Video 8.12. Apical four-chamber view showing an almost normal LVEF after discontinuation of traztuzumab. Simpson biplane LVEF is 50%

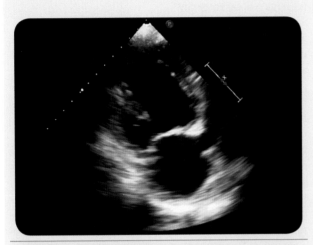

Video 8.13. Apical two-chamber view. See **Video 8.12**

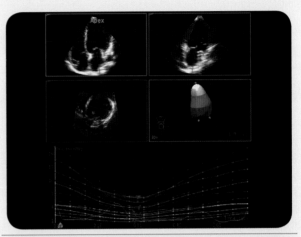

Video 8.14. Four-beats triggered full volume acquisition that enabled an accurate calculation of 3D-LVEF, which was 52%

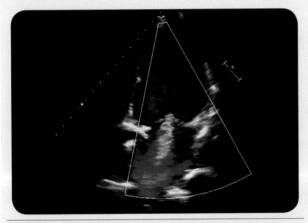

Video 8.15. Color-Doppler four-chamber view, where a persistent severe mitral regurgitation can be observed, in spite of the improvement in LVEF

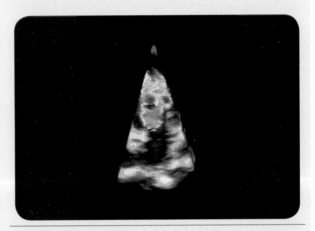

Video 8.16. 3D color full volume severe mitral regurgitation

Figures

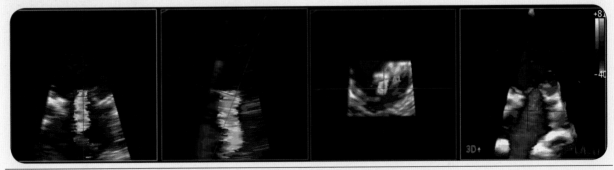

Figure 8.1. 3D-multiplanar reconstruction of the mitral regurgitating jet, which enables a direct measurement of the vena contr acta area of 0.52 cm², consistent with severe mitral regurgitation

8.2. Discussion

In this case we present a woman with a high-risk breast cancer, who requires multiple potentially cardiotoxic cancer treatments. During the first treatment she received epirrubicin, cyclophosphamide and paclitaxel combined with high dose radiotherapy, but cardiac evaluation was not performed at that time.

An echocardiography performed at the time of her first relapse showed a normal LVEF associated with grade II/IV valvular disease. Trastuzumab and doxorubicin in combination with lapatinib, taxol, carboplatin and gemcitabine were consecutively used in therapeutic schemes. The combined use of potentially cardiotoxic drugs increases the risk of cardiotoxicity, thus we are facing a high-risk situation.

At the time of her first relapse, the picture we meet is a middle-aged woman, with several cardiovascular risk factors (hypertension, and chronic kidney disease), previous anthracyclines use and mild mitral valve disease. These factors must be taken into account when assessing the risk/benefit ratio of a new cardiotoxic treatment. Although primary prevention with cardioprotective drugs is not yet universally recommended, it should be individually considered whenever there is a high probability of developing cardiotoxicity. In this case, where an aggressive anticancer treatment can be expected, due to the unfavorable course of the oncologic disease, the patient could have clearly benefited from an early introduction of ACEI and/or beta-blockers as primary prevention of cardiotoxicity.

In this case, several mechanisms are responsible for the cardiac dysfunction. Systolic function impairment is most likely secondary to the additive toxic effect of anthracyclines and trastuzumab, while mitral regurgitation is probably due to a combination of mitral valve thickening and calcification related to radiotherapy and functional mitral regurgitation.

When LV dysfunction was diagnosed, trastuzumab was held for two months; however, although LVEF did not fully recover, it did improve to almost normal values, and after careful consideration, it was restarted, as it was considered that the risk of her breast cancer progression was higher than the risk of heart failure, and trastuzumab is a cornerstone of chemotherapy in this particular case. Under treatment with ACEI and beta-blockers the patient has been doing well, with no heart failure signs or symptoms and stable LVEF to date.

8.3. Conclusions

Previous treatment with potentially cardiotoxic drugs increases the risk of developing cardiotoxicity. Early start of cardioprotective drugs could delay or even prevent the development of myocardial dysfunction whenever a new cardiotoxic treatment is required.

Case 09

Previous Cardiovascular Disease as a Risk Factor of Cardiotoxicity

Oscar González Fernández
Silvia Valbuena López

Cardiology Department. La Paz University Hospital. IdiPAz Research Institute. Madrid. Spain

9.1. Case Presentation

An 84-year-old white male was seen in the Emergency department because of dyspnea and edema in December 2013. The patient was a former smoker and had a history of diabetes and ischemic heart disease. He had an inferior acute ST elevation myocardial infarction in 2000, when a conventional balloon angioplasty of the right coronary artery was performed. Because of the presence of three-vessel diffuse coronary artery disease, a coronary artery bypass graft surgery was performed afterwards. He had been in his usual health until January 2012, when a mantle cell lymphoma was diagnosed. The lymphoma was a blastoid variant at stage IV-A, with a mantle cell lymphoma international prognostic index score of 6.5, considered as a high-risk lymphoma. Medications included aspirin, metformin, and sitagliptin.

An echocardiography performed before receiving any treatment revealed inferior wall akinesia with a LVEF of 52%, assessed with the biplane Simpson´s method **(Video 9.1, Video 9.2, Video 9.3, and Video 9.4).** The patient began an attenuated immuno-chemotherapy regimen (R-miniCHOP), which includes rituximab combined with low-dose cyclophosphamide, doxorubicin, vincristine, and prednisone at three-week intervals. Serial echocardiograms performed while receiving chemotherapy showed a slight decrease in LVEF. When treatment was completed, the patient had a LVEF of 45% and remained asymptomatic.

Six months after concluding treatment, a routine follow-up echocardiography revealed severe left ventricular systolic dysfunction. LVEF was 30%, and there was inferior wall akinesia and severe hypokinesia of the remaining segments **(Video 9.5 , Video 9.6, Video 9.7, and Video 8).** The patient had a NYHA functional class of II and treatment with bisoprolol, enalapril, and eplerenone was initiated.

Three months later (December 2013) the patient was seen in the Emergency department after developing heart failure symptoms. He reported minimal activity dyspnea during the week before. On examination blood pressure was 132/63 mmHg, heart rate was 67 bpm, temperature was 36 ºC and oxygen saturation was 94% while he was breathing ambient air. Carotid pulse and jugular veins were normal. Heart sounds had a regular rhythm without murmurs. He had crackles over the lower third of the right lung field and lower limb edema. The remainder of the examination was normal.

An electrocardiogram revealed sinus rhythm at a rate of 65 bpm with no other abnormalities. A chest X-ray showed cardiomegaly, cephalization of the pulmonary vessels and Kerley B-lines without pleural effusion. Blood test showed hemoglobin 11.9 g/dL, hematocrit 34.9%, white-cell count 5,300/mL with a normal percentage of band forms (61.6%), platelet count of 118,000/mL. Sodium, potassium, chloride, glucose, creatinine, and C-reactive protein were normal. NT-proBNP levels were 25,873 pg/dL.

The patient could be discharged after 24-hours of intravenous furosemide treatment, adding oral furosemide to his usual medication. No more episodes of acute decompensated heart failure or lymphoma recurrences occurred over the next 12 months. The patient undergoes regular follow-up with LVEF 33% in spite of optimal medical therapy.

Videos

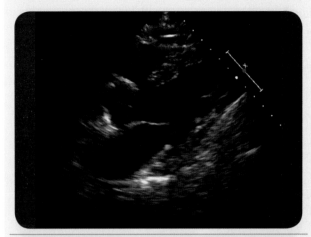

Video 9.1. Parasternal long-axis view showing normal mitral and aortic valves with lower limit value of left ventricular function

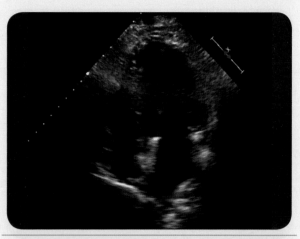

Video 9.2. Apical four-chamber view showing lower limit value of left ventricular function

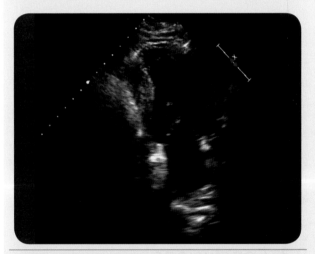

Video 9.3. Apical two-chamber view showing inferior wall akinesia. See **Video 9.2**

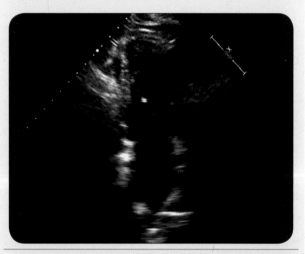

Video 9.4. Apical three-chamber view showing lower limit value of left ventricular function. See **Video 9.2**

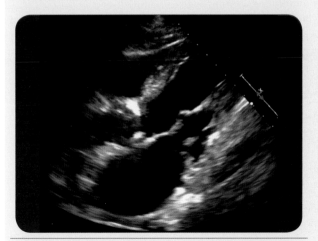

Video 9.5. Parasternal long-axis view showing normal mitral and aortic valves with dilated left ventricle and severe systolic dysfunction

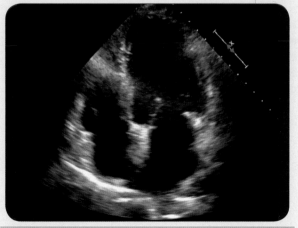

Video 9.6. Apical four-chamber view showing severe left ventricular dysfunction

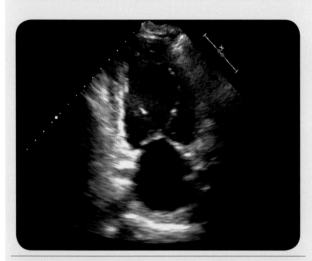

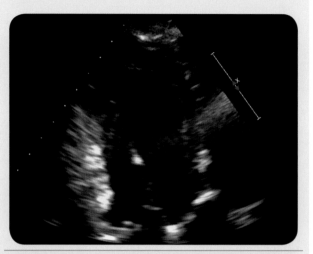

Video 9.7. Apical two-chamber view. See **Video 9.6**

Video 9.8. Apical three-chamber view. See **Video 9.6**

9.2. Discussion

This clinical case illustrates the development of left ventricular systolic dysfunction after chemotherapy in a patient with previous ischemic heart disease. Anthracycline therapy is well known as a potential cause of cardiotoxicity and most lymphoma chemotherapy regimens include these drugs. Some risk factors for the development of chronic anthracycline cardiotoxicity have been identified. Cumulative dose is considered the strongest predictor of cardiotoxicity. However, age, concomitant cardiotoxic chemotherapy agents, concurrent or prior radiation therapy, and pre-existing cardiovascular disease are also well-known risk factors.

Monitoring of cardiac function before, during, and after treatment is highly recommended in patients undergoing anthracycline-containing chemotherapy. LVEF should be periodically evaluated, echocardiography being the standard approach for its evaluation. The use of troponins or deformation parameters in echocardiography like GLS may give an early indication of cardiac damage.

The most important message in cardiotoxicity prevention is the need for close collaboration between hematologists and cardiologists to avoid serious complications in high risk patients (advanced age, diabetes, previous ischemic heart disease and LVEF in the low range of normal). The primary prevention of cardiotoxicity is still a matter of controversy today. However, our patient was already in stage B of heart failure, and the optimization of cardiovascular treatment, with beta-blockers and ACEIs, is essential to minimize anthracycline cardiotoxicity.

9.3. Conclusions

Anthracyclines are some of the most frequently implicated agents in cardiotoxicity. Cumulative dose, age, and pre-existing cardiovascular disease have been identified as main risk factors for anthracycline-related cardiotoxicity. Optimization of heart failure treatment and multidiciplinary cardio-oncologic teams are mandatory to reduce cancer therapeutic-related cardiac disease.

Case 10

Use of Cardiac Biomarkers in the Follow-up of an Oncologic Patient

Afonso Freitas Ferraz
Alberto Cecconi

Cardiology Department. San Carlos University Hospital. Madrid. Spain

10.1. Case Presentation

We present the case of a 59-year-old male, former smoker, with a history of dyslipidemia, a cytomegalovirus hepatitis, and a post-traumatic pneumothorax after a car accident during his youth.

Following a conjuntival biopsy of the right eye, the patient was diagnosed with diffuse large B-cell lymphoma (DLBCL), stage IV, with ocular, dorso-lumbar spine and epidural invasion and International Prognostic Index (IPI) = 3 (stage IV, extranodal site > 1 and increased serum LDH levels).

Due to the good initial response after receiving radiotherapy over the lumbar spine (five sessions), chemotherapy with rituximab + cyclophosphamide + doxorubicin + vincristine + prednisolone was administered every 14 days (R-CHOP/14) for six cycles; central nervous system prophylaxis with methotrexate was added to the treatment, thus achieving complete remission.

Before the first cycle of chemotherapy, in order to establish baseline parameters to serve as reference in subsequent reviews, a number of cardiologic tests were performed including: echocardiography assessment of the LVEF in 2D **(Video 10.1)** and 3D **(Video 10.2)**; GLS **(Figure 10.1)** and high-sensitivity troponin I and T serum levels. **Table 10.1** shows the evolution of these parameters and their temporal relationship with chemotherapy regimens. In tests taken at the third month, coinciding with the last cycle of R-CHOP/14, we observed an increase in high-sensitivity troponin I and T serum levels and a mild decline in GLS with no change in LVEF **(Figure 10.2).** This trend con-

tinued till the sixth month, with the patient remaining asymptomatic from the cardiovascular standpoint. Finally, 12 months after starting chemotherapy, an evident decrease in LVEF begins with troponin levels that continue slightly elevated and a more pronounced decrease in GLS **(Video 10.3).** After a careful cardiologic evaluation, treatment with beta-blockers and ACEI was promptly initiated, although they had to be eventually discontinued due to persistent symptomatic hypotension.

A few days later, a recurrence in the central nervous system was diagnosed and a new chemotherapy regimen was commenced: rituximab + etoposide + methylprednisolone + cytarabine + cisplatin (R-ESHAP).

During clinical follow-up the patient showed signs and symptoms of functional class deterioration (NYHA II-III) and persistent mild left ventricular dysfunction in echocardiography monitoring; hence, beta-blockers were reinstated at a lower dose with no further adverse effects. Two months after the last cycle of R-ESHAP, after which complete remission was achieved, the patient underwent conditioning regimen with BEAM (carmustine + etoposide + cytarabine + mephalan) followed by an autologous hematopoietic cell transplantation (AHCT). The patient presented gastrointestinal and hepatic toxicity, and febrile neutropenia as side effects.

Despite the good initial response, a few months later the patient presented with vomiting and blurred vision and central nervous system involvement was confirmed by the presence of tumor cells in cerebrospinal fluid cytology. The patient underwent salvage therapy with intrathecal rituximab and a conditioned regimen with BAM (high dose of methotrexate + cytarabine +

carmustine) aiming at a second AHCT. Nevertheless, a brain MRI showed intraventricular ependymal nodules enhancement suggesting brain metastases. Given the extent of the disease and its refractoriness to multiple lines of CT regimens, it was decided to withhold further treatment and prioritize palliative care. The patient died three years after the initial diagnosis.

Videos

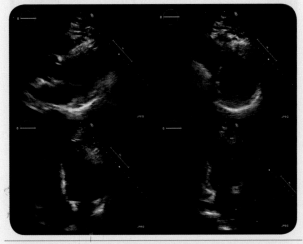

Video 10.1. Baseline TTE. 2D-views showing normal left ventricular function. LVEF was measured in 63%

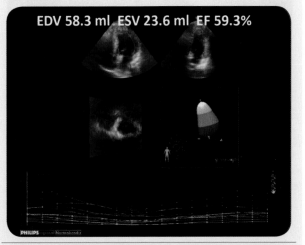

Video 10.2. Baseline TTE. 3D-analysis shows LVEF 59%

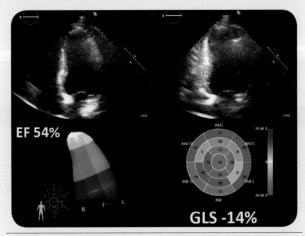

Video 10.3. A 12 months TTE evaluation. GLS has decreased to -14% and LVEF is 53%, 10% less than basal evaluation

Figures

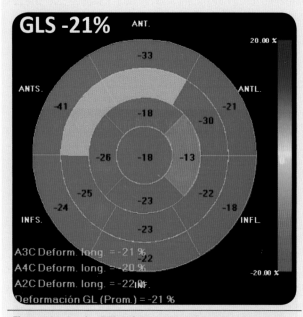

Figure 10.1. Baseline TTE. GLS was measured in -21%

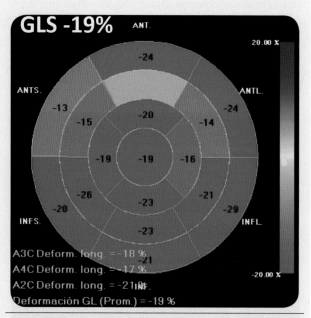

Figure 10.2. Three months follow-up GLS

Tables

	Baseline	21 days	3 months	6 months	12 months	18 months	24 months	30 months
LVEF 2D (%)	63		68	57	53	49*	48	57
LVEF 3D (%)	59		64		54	*		
GLS (%)	-21		-19	-18	-14	*		
Hs-cTnT* (pg/mL)	9.74	14	44.87	18.55	17.55	19.6	19.63	
Hs-cTnI** (pg/mL)	3.6	4.9	58.6	14.9	10.2	7.1	9	

* Cut-off value hs-cTnT 14 pg/mL
** Cut-off value hs-cTnI 26.2 pg/mL
* Poor acoustic window. Other echocardiographic parameters could not be established. LVEF confirmed by cardiac MRI

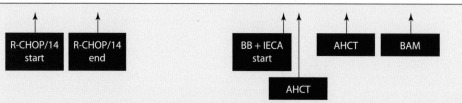

Table 10.1. Time course of ventricular function, high-sensitivity troponin levels and their temporal relationship with chemotherapy regimens

10.2. Discussion

Diffuse large B cell lymphoma is the most common histologic subtype, accounting for 30% to 58% of non-Hodgkin lymphoma cases. As in most cases (60%) of diffuse large B cell lymphoma, our patient was diagnosed at an advanced stage (III and IV) of the disease. For patients treated with R-CHOP, an IPI = 3 predicts a survival rate of approximately 57% at four years, which places our patient within a group of intermediate-high risk.

Regimens containing anthracyclines, such as R-CHOP, are a mainstay in this group of patients, where it demonstrated increased survival. As a result, we face an ever-growing number of long-term cancer survivors suffering from comorbidities related to cytostatic agents. Within this group, cardiotoxicity has become the leading cause of morbidity and mortality and is a common complication of many anti-tumoral agents that may compromise clinical effectiveness of chemotherapy.

The incidence of anthracycline cardiotoxicity is 4% to > 36%. In this case, some factors that may have increased the risk are the cumulative dose and the use of other cardiotoxic agents such as cyclophosphamide.

The actual definition of cardiotoxicity establishes LVEF as the decisive factor, so that a reduction in LVEF from baseline ≥ 10% to < 53% establishes the diagnosis. One of the major limitations of this definition is the inherent technique variability in the measurement of LVEF and the fact that the reduction of LVEF is a late phenomenon, limiting the use of this criterion in clinical practice. Hence, it is necessary to establish a diagnostic method for predicting early the development of cardiotoxicity and thus allowing treatment to be initiated promptly.

In line with this argument, a fall in GLS > 15% from basal value has proven to be an earlier predictor of cardiotoxicity with less inter and intra-observer variability. In our case **(Table 10.1),** the GLS showed an early reduction of 14% at six months (from -21% to -18%) compared to the later decrease in LVEF that was only clinically significant at 12 months.

Likewise, identification of biomarkers able to specifically detect myocardial injury, namely troponins levels, have been shown in several studies to be very early predictors of chemotherapy-induced cardiotoxicity.

Patients with a persistent troponin I elevation one month after treatment with chemotherapy were at the greatest risk of cardiac events which included: sudden death, cardiovascular mortality, asymptomatic ventricular dysfunction, heart failure, malignant arrhythmias, and pacemaker implantation. In contrast, patients with only a transient elevation had a much lower incidence of cardiac events (37% *versus* 84%).

Our patient belongs to the highest risk group, with persistently elevated troponin. In previous studies, over 80% of patients with this profile elevation develops some degree of left ventricular systolic dysfunction. Previous studies have found that early treatment with ACEI in patients with elevated troponin I (one month after the last dose of CT) prevents cardiotoxicity and improves cardiologic outcome when compared to those untreated.

10.3. Conclusions

The monitoring of patients by classical methods based on the quantification of LVEF has a low sensitivity to predict myocardial injury, which determines a late diagnosis and treatment. Measurement of high-sensitivity troponins and GLS may become a useful routine method for identifying patients more prone to developing cardiotoxicity and in whom a preventive pharmacologic strategy and closer cardiac monitoring are imperative.

Case 11

Development of Left Ventricular Dysfunction after Rechallenge with Cardiotoxic Drugs

Juan Caro Codón
Sandra Rosillo Rodríguez

Cardiology Department. La Paz University Hospital. IdiPAz Research Institute. Madrid. Spain

11.1. Case Presentation

We present the case of a 51-year-old woman, with dyslipidemia as the only cardiovascular risk factor who, ten years ago, was diagnosed with infiltrating ductal carcinoma of the right breast, pT3pN2a. Pathologic analyses were positive for hormone receptors and HER2. She received neoadjuvant chemotherapy with epirubicin and docetaxel and subsequently underwent surgical tumorectomy and lymphadenectomy. She later received six cycles of adjuvant chemotherapy (including cyclophosphamide, epirubicin, and 5-fluorouracil). Hormonal therapy with anastrazol was maintained for five years.

A total of 10 years later, after being diagnosed with local recurrence, a biopsy revealed a multicentric tumor, pT1b G1 and pT1b pleomorfic G3, with hormone receptors present but negative for HER2. Total mastectomy was performed. Prior to the start of adjuvant chemotherapy, a transthoracic echocardiography was performed, which showed normal systolic function (left ventricular ejection fraction, LVEF, 56%), without regional wall motion abnormalities **(Video 11.1 and Video 11.2)**. Paclitaxel and doxorubicin (total doses: 400 mg) were initiated.

The patient underwent irregular cardiac surveillance and 12 months after the start of chemotherapy a transthoracic echocardiography revealed global hypokinesis, with moderate left ventricular dysfunction (LVEF 43% and GLS of -14%) and moderate mitral regurgitation **(Video 11.3, Video 11.4, Video 11.5, and Figure 11.1)**. Estimated pulmonary artery systolic pressure was 50 mmHg. Treatment with ACEI and beta-blockers was initiated but, despite initial clinical improvement, she progressively developed moderate-to-severe heart failure symptoms. Subsequent decline of left ventricular systolic function was documented with echocardiography, which showed severe left ventricular dysfunction with an estimated LVEF of 31% and a GLS of -11% **(Figure 11.2 and Video 11.6)**. Cardiac treatment was reinforced with aldosterone antagonists. Despite optimal dosage of these drugs, moderate left ventricular dysfunction (LVEF 38%) persisted in serial echocardiography after a six-month follow-up. Nevertheless, the patient has been doing well from a clinical point of view, and is currently free of heart failure symptoms.

Videos

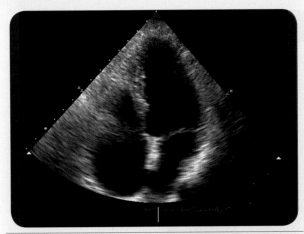

Video 11.1. Apical four-chamber view showed preserved LVEF without regional wall motion abnormalities

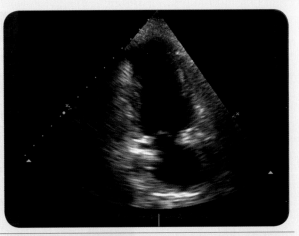

Video 11.2. Apical two-chamber view showing normal contractility

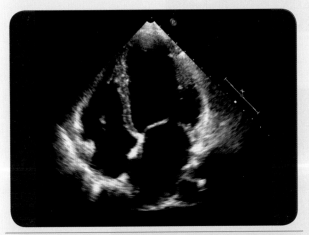

Video 11.3. Apical four-chamber view showed global hypokinesis with moderate depression of LV contractility

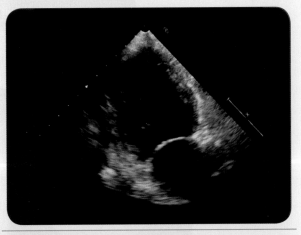

Video 11.4. Apical two-chamber view confirmed moderate left ventricular systolic dysfunction

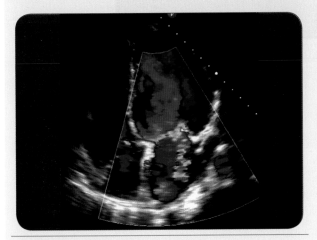

Video 11.5. Color-Doppler apical four-chamber view shows a moderate mitral regurgitation

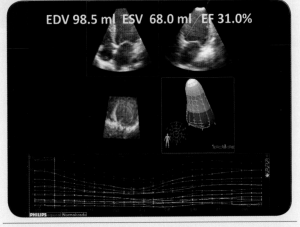

Video 11.6. 3D-analysis revealed severe left ventricular contractility dysfunction

Figures

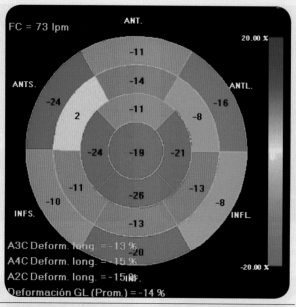

Figure 11.1. Bull's eye view of global longitudinal strain analysis reveals marked abnormalities in deformation parameters (GLS -14%)

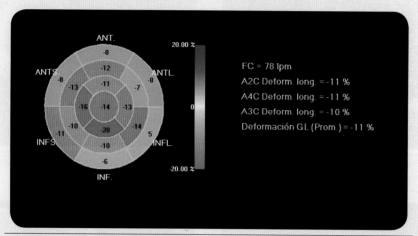

Figure 11.2. The patient not only suffered marked depression in LVEF but also had subsequent deterioration of GLS

11.2. Discussion

Anthracycline and, in particular, doxorubicin toxicity is mediated by the formation of ternary complexes with toposisomerase-IIβ and deoxyribonucleic acid, which are responsible for mitochondrial alterations and oxidative stress. This results in ultraestructural changes and, ultimately, cell death.

Dose-dependent cardiac toxicity limits the use of anthracyclines in the management of oncologic patients. Therefore, different strategies have been attempted to prevent the development of ventricular dysfunction in these patients, such as limiting the cumulative dose of administered anthracyclines as much as possible (ideally below 450 mg/m^2 of doxorubicin), continuous intravenous infusions and the use of liposomal doxorrubicin.

This case illustrates the importance of close clinical and echocardiographic follow-up in this group of patients, which should be included in a multidisciplinary management protocol that includes scheduled cardiac surveillance. Early detection of myocardial dysfunction is crucial, as reversibility of the toxicity is directly related to the time to diagnosis, with very low rates of LVEF recovery if this delay is over six months. This is especially impor-tant in the population of patients with previous treatment with anthracyclines, as they may already have subclinical myocardial damage.

In our case, considering the patient's medical history, closer follow-up should have been performed. In an optimal environment, the use of cardiac biomarkers and myocardial deformation techniques would be desirable, as they improve the diagnosis of myocardial toxicity.

11.3. Conclusions

This case report illustrates that patients previously treated with anthracyclines who need to be rechallenged with this type of antineoplastic drugs, might already have a subclinical myocardial damage, undetectable for standard echocardiography. This condition places them at higher risk of developing cancer therapeutic-related cardiac damage, so preventive strategies should be emphasized, and their inclusion in a multidisciplinary follow-up program, including cardiologists with expertise in the care of cancer patients, is strongly recommended.

Case 12

Symptomatic Sinus Tachycardia during Chemotherapy; Association with Overall Cardiac Mortality

Sandra Rosillo Rodríguez
Juan Caro Codón

Cardiology Department. La Paz University Hospital. IdiPAz Research Institute. Madrid. Spain

12.1. Case Presentation

A 37-year-old women with no previous medical history, presented to the hospital complaining of 15 days of moderate exertional dyspnea, palpitations, dry postural cough, night sweating, and marked edema of the face and upper body. In the physical examination there was an outstanding fixed erythema and swelling of the face, superior thorax and upper extremities which worsened by squatting and in the zero degree decubitus position. Extensive thoracic collateral circulation and jugular vein distention that did not collapse during inspiration were both also present. Blood tests were normal. A chest X-ray supported the presence of a widened mediastinum and normal-sized heart cavities. Electrocardiogram was consistent with sinus tachycardia (120 bpm) with no other associated conduction or repolarization abnormalities. Echocardiographic parameters were found to be within normal range. The 2D-LVEF with the Simpson biplane method was 67% **(Video 12.1, Video 12.2, and Video 12.3)**; 3D-LVEF was 60% **(Video 12.4)** and GLS showed a normal value (-23.7%; **Figure 12.1).**

With the clinical diagnosis of a superior vena cava syndrome, a CT scan was scheduled in order to try to determine the etiol-

ogy. It revealed the presence of an 8 x 7 x 6 cm heterogeneous and hypointense mass that contacted with the ascending aorta, left bronquius, as well as left pulmonary veins and left pulmonary artery. The superior vena cava was completely collapsed by this mass **(Figure 12.2).** A guided percutaneous biopsy was performed, being compatible with a diffuse large B-cell non-Hodgkin lymphoma.

Afterwards, a front-line chemotherapeutic regimen under the denomination EPOCH-R (etoposide, prednisone, vincristine, cyclophosphamide, doxorubicin, and rituximab) was established, with acceptable tolerance and scarce adverse events, except for the development of peripheral neuropathy treated successfully with amitriptyline and vitamin B.

From a cardiologic point of view, the patient complains of slight deterioration in functional class along with an unexplained persistent sinus tachycardia after the first chemotherapy cycle. She was referred for cardiac evaluation. We found no significant changes in ejection fraction. 2D-ejection fraction at three-month follow-up was 59% and global longitudinal strain was -20.2% **(Figure 12.3).** We started on beta-blockers (bisoprolol 2.5 mg/day), with improvement in symptoms and the heart rate up to normal levels. At one-year follow-up clinical course was uneventful.

Videos

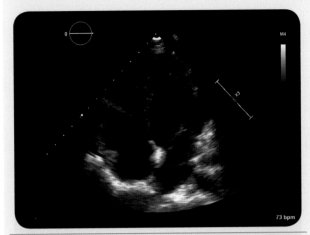

Video 12.1. Normal transthoracic echocardiography in apical four-chamber view. On the left of the image we can see an abnormal extracardiac structure corresponding with tumoral mass

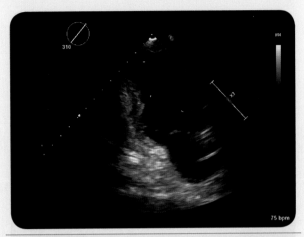

Video 12.2. Normal transthoracic echocardiography in apical two-chamber view

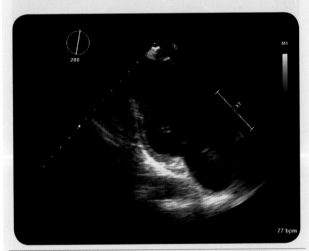

Video 12.3. Normal transthoracic echocardiography in apical three-chamber view

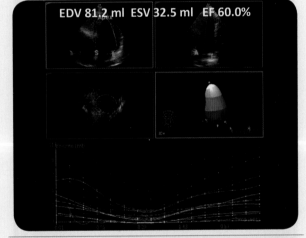

Video 12.4. 3D quantification of left ventricular ejection fraction

Figures

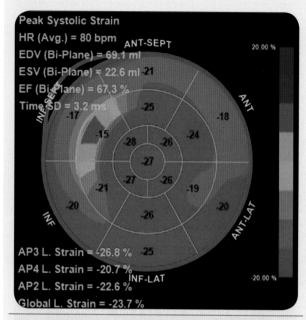

Figure 12.1. Baseline quantification of global longitudinal strain

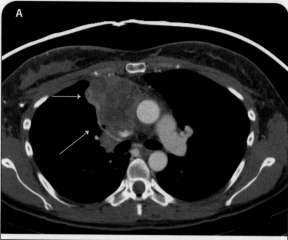

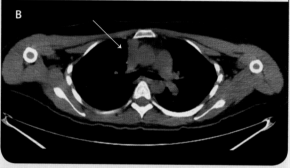

Figure 12.2. CT scan evaluation. **A:** baseline showing the presence of a mediastinal mass compressing the superior vena cava; **B:** five months after the beginning of the chemotherapeutic treatment, showing a reduction of more than 50% of the initial reported diameter of the mass

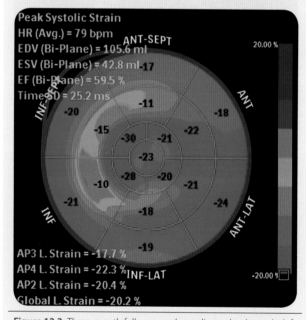

Figure 12.3. Three-month follow-up echocardiography showed a left ventricular ejection fraction of 59% and global longitudinal strain of -20.2%

12.2. Discussion

Heart rate is a very accessible clinical variable and numerous studies performed throughout the past 20 years in the general population and particularly in patients with different burdens of cardiovascular disease including hypertension, acute myocardial infarction, heart failure, or left ventricular dysfunction, have found a significant association between elevated resting heart rate and all-cause cardiovascular mortality, which is independent from other demographic or clinical variables.

Moreover, heart rate has been associated with scarce exercise capacity, which is a powerful predictor of mortality and it is also the common denominator in metabolic syndrome (hypertension, atherogenic lipid profile, insulin resistance, and overweight) which also entails cardiovascular mortality.

Beta-blockers through their negative chronotropic effect have proven to reduce mortality in both ischemic heart disease and heart failure patients; the best prognosis was observed in patients with lowest baseline heart rate and the greatest heart rate reduction after initiation of therapy.

As nowadays there is still a lack of consensus on the establishment of primary preventive therapies (including beta-blockers or ACEI) in patients at high-risk of developing cardiotoxicity (stage A of the AHA/ACC heart failure classification), the appearance of a symptomatic sinus tachycardia is probably the best scenario for beginning beta-blocker therapy, which on the other hand is already showing its beneficial effects (OVERCOME trial: prevention of left ventricular dysfunction with enalapril and carvedilol in patients submitted to intensive chemotherapy for the treatment of hemopathies).

12.3. Conclusions

Elevated heart rate is an independent variable for all-cause cardiovascular mortality. Beta-blockers have proven to increase survival in heart failure patients. Considering the fact that exposure to cardiotoxic drugs is stage A of heart failure, as recognized by the AHA/ACC guidelines, studies are being performed to try to establish a formal indication for the initiation of beta-blockers as primary prevention drugs in this population. In case of observed unexplained sinus tachycardia in the follow-up of patients undergoing cardiotoxic chemotherapy, beta-blockers are highly recommended.

Case 13

Cardiotoxicity Monitorization during Chemotherapy

Carlos Ferrera Durán
Afonso Freitas Ferraz

Cardiology Department. San Carlos University Hospital. Madrid. Spain

13.1. Case Presentation

A 29-year-old obese man came to hospital because of sore throat, shivering, constipation, and abdominal pain located in the left hypochondrium. He had no history of previous cardiopathy or cardiovascular risk factors. Physical examination revealed a temperature of 37.7 ºC, and presence of multiple left latero-cervical and supra-clavicular lymphadenopathies. Blood analysis showed a severe lecukocytosis (129 x 10⁹/L), predominantly lymphocytes, and presence of blasts (60%), as well as anemia (Hb 13.5 g/L), and thrombocytopenia (85,000 platelets/L). Under suspicion of acute myeloid leukemia the patient was admitted to hospital. Hydration and cyto-reduction therapy with hydroxyurea and tumor-lysis prophylaxis was immediately initiated. Bone marrow aspirate confirmed diagnosis of acute myeloid leukemia with monocyte origin.

After diagnosis and prior to chemotherapy initiation, a transthoracic echocardiography was performed, showing both ventricles with normal dimension without regional wall motion abnormalities. LVEF measured by Simpson biplane method (57%) and 3D-method (57%) was also normal **(Video 13.1 and Video 13.2)**; right systolic function (TAPSE 23 mm) was normal too. Speckle tracking assessment showed a GLS of -17.5% **(Video 13.3).** Diastolic function parameters were also within normal range (E/A ratio 1.2, and E/E' ration 10.7). Transthoracic echocardiography also found a bicuspid but functionally normal aortic valve and aortic root dilation (40 mm).

After transthoracic echocardiography, an initial cycle of chemotherapy with idarubicin (26.76 mg) for three days plus cytarabine (446 mg) as continuous infusion for seven days was administered. The patient developed febrile neutropenia, abdominal pain, and diarrhea that resolved after correct hydration and antibiotic therapy. Control bone marrow aspirate found minimal residual disease of 1.2%. Control transthoracic echocardiography after the first cycle of chemotherapy showed no significant changes with respect to baseline echo (LVEF 57%, GLS -17%, and normal right ventricular function).

A new control bone marrow that showed a residual disease of 3% was performed one week later. A new chemotherapy cycle with idarubicin (27.77 mg) for three days plus cytarabine (412.8 mg) as continuous infusion for seven days was administered and well tolerated. However, bone marrow aspiration after this cycle again revealed residual disease of 3.7%. Given the high-risk of the patient, rescue therapy with ICE (idarubicin 25.92 mg for two days + citarabin 4,320 mg bid for two days, and etoposide 216 mg for two days) was scheduled and followed by bone marrow transplantation. The patient was then treated with immunosuppressants (cyclosporine, mycofenolat mofetil). A transthoracic echocardiography was performed just after the third cycle of chemotherapy. A drop in deformation parameters with strain assessment (GLS -14.8%) was found, while LVEF with the Simpson method (53%) and 3D-method (59%) remained within normal limits. Given these findings, a new transthoracic echocardiography study was scheduled two weeks after chemotherapy, in order to confirm the abnormalities in deformation parameters.

Transthoracic echocardiography study after two weeks confirmed the drop in GLS (-13.4%) but the LVEF remained stable by both the Simpson biplane method (54%) and 3D-method (57%).

(Video 13.4, Video 13.5, and Figure 13.1). Carvedilol treatment was commenced. However, durant immunosuppressant therapy the patient developed hypertension and hypercholesterolemia as a complication of cyclosporine, which was appropri-ately controlled with statins, ACEI and beta-blockers permitting the patient to complete the scheduled hematologic treatment. Two months after completion of chemotherapy the patient was stable and asymptomatic under cardiac treatment.

Videos

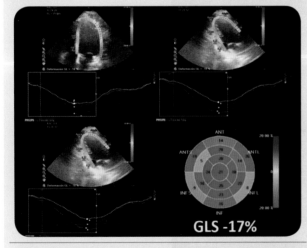

Video 13.1. Baseline transthoracic echocardiography evaluation before chemotherapy. The video shows normal left ventricular function

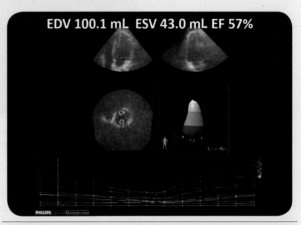

Video 13.2. 3D-view in the baseline transesophagic echocardiography for accurate measurements of left ventricular end-systolic and end-diastolic volumes and LVEF

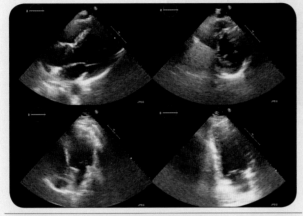

Video 13.3. GLS before chemotherapy. The baseline value was -17.5%

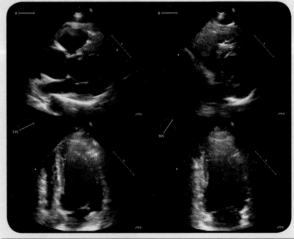

Video 13.4. Transthoracic echocardiography evaluation after three cycles of chemotherapy, where apparently normal left ventricular function can be observed

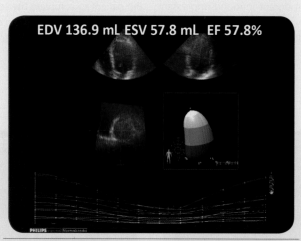

Video 13.5. 3D-view in transthoracic echocardiography after chemotherapy displays a normal value of LVEF (56%)

Figures

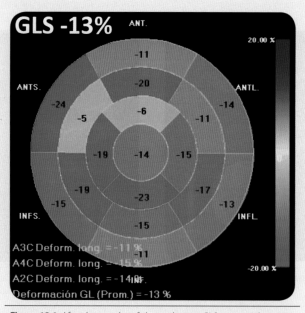

Figure 13.1. After three cycles of chemotherapy GLS worsened to -13%

13.2. Discussion

This case is a good example of early detection of cardiotoxicity secondary to chemotherapy with anthracyclines in a patient with acute myeloid leukemia. Anthracyclines are high-effective chemotherapy agents, whose use is still widespread in the therapy against many types of cancer. Endomyocardial biopsy studies and myocardial markers such as troponins measurements suggest that myocyte damage may occur during treatment or early after exposure to anthracyclines. However, clinical manifestations could not become apparent until months to years after the initial exposure.

The incidence of anthracycline-related cardiotoxicity is dose-dependent and varies between 2.2 to 5.1%. The mechanism of anthracycline cardiotoxicity is complex and not fully understood. Anthracyclines must enter the myocytes to cause damage. Once inside the cell, the drug induces the formation of reactive oxygen species and mitochondrial dysfunction, and consequently changes in calcium homeostasis and contractile function. Furthermore increase of drug concentration inside the cell causes myocyte death by apoptosis and necrosis.

The guidelines from the *European Society of Cardiology* recommend a complete medical history, physical examination, blood analysis with cardiac biomarkers measurement, an electrocardiogram, and an echocardiography with assessment of left ventricular function prior to administration of chemotherapy.

Transthoracic echocardiography is the imaging modality of choice for initial and follow-up assessment of cardiac function during therapy with cardiotoxic agents. The current definition of cardiotoxicity is based on a reduction in LVEF > 10% and lower than 53%. Cardiotoxicity can be further classified as symptomatic or asymptomatic and as reversible or non-reversible depending on patient clinical course. Despite widespread use, LVEF is much less than perfect for evaluation of oncologic patients. First, there are technical issues because measurement variability can be higher than thresholds used to define cardiotoxicity. More important is the fact that reduction in LVEF is a late phenomenon, with failure to recover systolic function in up to 58% of patients despite intervention.

Myocardial deformation evaluation has been shown to be able to detect early subclinical ventricular dysfunction before LVEF reduction. A relative reduction of GLS > 15% from patient basal value is predictive of development of cardiotoxicity in the follow-up. Abnormal GLS value enables an early introduction of cardiac therapy that has critical clinical value. Statins, beta-blockers, and ACEI should be initiated whereas calcium channel blockers have no shown benefit in this context.

Our patient had -17.5% at baseline and experienced a drop up to a value of -13.4% after three cycles of anthracyclines. It is worth pointing out the importance of using each patient as their own control, leading to potential variability in the different measurements. In accordance with previous studies, our patient maintained LVEF within normal range, despite deterioration in deformation parameters. In those patients with significant reduction of LVEF or GLS, a new transthoracic echocardiography after two weeks is recommended for confirmation of the findings. If the alteration is confirmed, discussion with the oncologist is warranted to assess therapeutic strategy.

13.3. Conclusions

Echocardiography is the technique of choice for monitorization of heart structure and function during treatment with cardiotoxic agents. GLS allows us to early detect subclinical impairment in left ventricular systolic function during chemotherapy and identify patients who benefit from early cardio-protective intervention.

Case 14

Transient Anthracycline-Induced Left Ventricular Dysfunction

Sandra Rosillo Rodríguez
Juan Caro Codón

Cardiology Department. La Paz University Hospital. IdiPAz Research Institute. Madrid. Spain

14.1. Case Presentation

A 40-year-old male with no previous medical history, presented to the hospital with a large palpable abdominal mass. After the performance of a directed biopsy, he was diagnosed with a non-Hodgkin B-cell follicular lymphoma which quickly transformed into a high grade diffuse large B-cell lymphoma with infiltration of the bone marrow, as well as dissemination to supra- and infra-diaphragmatic lymph nodes and peritoneum.

A front-line chemotherapeutic regimen for aggressive non-Hodgkin's lymphoma under the denomination EPOCH-R (etoposide, prednisone, vincristine, cyclophosphamide, doxorubicin, and rituximab) was established. Following a standardized protocol for early detection of cardiotoxicity in oncologic populations, the patient completed a full cardiologic assessment prior to beginning such a therapy. He was clinically asymptomatic, the electrocardiogram revealed a normal sinus rhythm with no associated conduction or repolarization abnormalities **(Figure 14.1)** and the echocardiographic parameters analyzed were within normal range including a 2D-LVEF of 64% **(Video 14.1, Video 14.2, and Video 14.3)**, a 3D-ejection fraction of 67% **(Video 14.4)** and a GLS of -22% **(Figure 14.2A).** After the third week of chemotherapy a significant fall in the GLS (-15%) was observed **(Figure 14.2B),** yet with preserved left ventricular ejection fraction (2D-LVEF of 58%).

At the end of the fifth cycle of chemotherapy, a control electrocardiogram showed a long QT corrected interval **(Figure 14.3)** and a transthoracic echocardiography detected moderate left ventricular dysfunction, with an estimated 2D-LVEF of 39% **(Video 14.5, Video 14.6, and Video 14.7)** and a 3D-ejection fraction of 37% **(Video 14.8)** and a GLS of -12.3% **(Figure 14.4);** which was otherwise asymptomatic. The evaluation was then completed by performing a cardiac magnetic resonance which ruled out the presence of edema, perfusion defects or pathologic late gadolinium enhancement; structural causes of left ventricular dysfunction were excluded and the diagnosis of anthracycline´s cardiac toxicity favored.

Bisoprolol, ramipril, and eplerenone were started and the patient underwent his sixth cycle of chemotherapy; anthracyclines were withdrawn from the regimen. After four weeks, a control transthoracic echocardiography demonstrated normalization of left ventricular ejection fraction (2D-LVEF 52%; 3D-LVEF 53%; GLS -16.5%) **(Video 14.9, Video 14.10, Video 14.11, Video 14.12, Video 14.13, and Figure 14.5).**

On the other hand, the follow-up PET-CT scan showed tumoral progression. At this point, a risk-benefit decision was made to expose the patient to a Hyper-CVAD (cyclophosphamide, vincristine, doxorubicin, and dexamethasone) regimen, even under the knowledge of the above described precedents and with sustained use of the cardio-protective drugs. After completion of chemotherapy the patient did not develop further cardiac complications.

Unfortunately, there was no tumoral response; at last an allogenic bone marrow transplant from the patient´s brother was at last performed. The patient continued to deteriorate and died three weeks after the transplant.

Videos

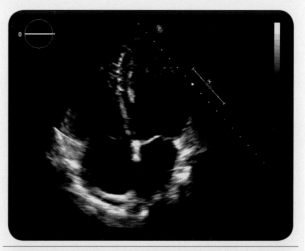

Video 14.1. Baseline 2D-echocardiography. Long-axis view

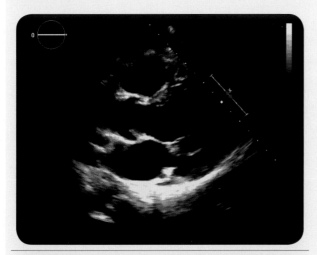

Video 14.2. Baseline 2D-echocardiography. Apical four-chamber view

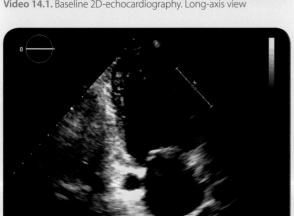

Video 14.3. Baseline 2D-echocardiography. Apical two-chamber view. 2D Simpson biplane 2D-left ventricular ejection fraction of 64%

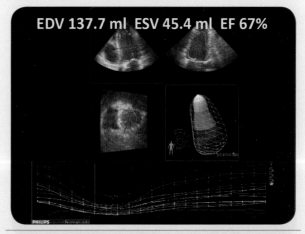

EDV 137.7 ml ESV 45.4 ml EF 67%

Video 14.4. Baseline 3D quantification of left ventricular. 3D-LVEF 67% ejection fraction

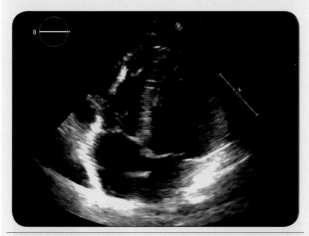

Video 14.5. 2D-transthoracic echocardiography performed at the end of the fifth cycle of chemotherapy. Four-chamber view

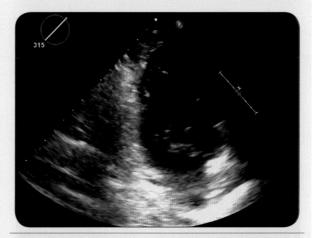

Video 14.6. 2D-transthoracic echocardiography performed at the end of the fifth cycle of chemotherapy. 2D Simpson biplane estimated 2D-left ventricular ejection fraction of 39%

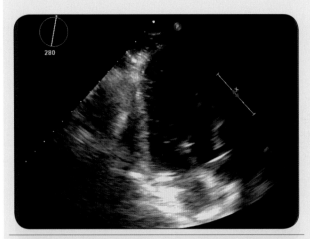

Video 14.7. 2D-transthoracic echocardiography performed at the end of the fifth cycle of chemotherapy. Three-chamber view

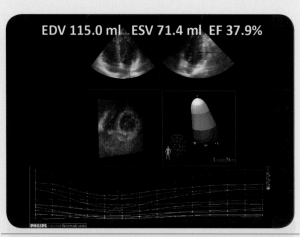

EDV 115.0 ml ESV 71.4 ml EF 37.9%

Video 14.8. 3D quantification of left ventricular ejection fraction performed at the end of the fifth cycle of chemotherapy (3D-LVEF 37%)

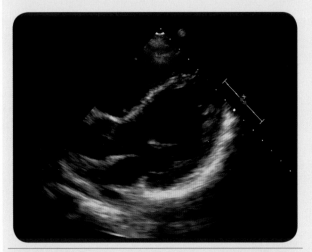

Video 14.9. After heart failure treatment a 2D-echo showed an improvement in 2D-LVEF. Parasternal long-axis view

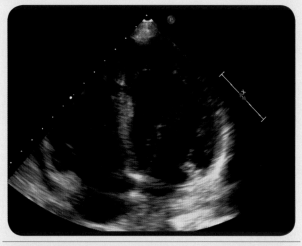

Video 14.10. 2D-transthoracic echocardiography performed after heart failure treatment. Apical four-chamber view

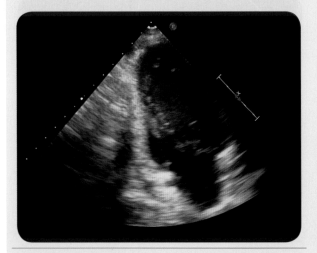

Video 14.11. 2D-transthoracic echocardiography performed after heart failure treatment. Apical two-chamber view. 2D-LVEF 52%

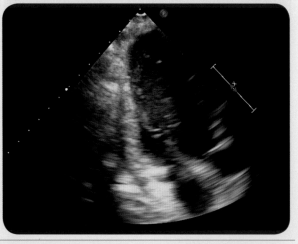

Video 14.12. 2D-transthoracic echocardiography performed after heart failure treatment. Apical three-chamber view

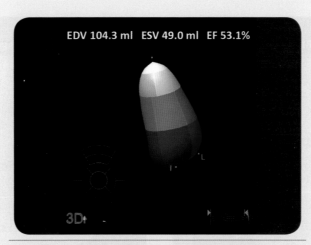

Video 14.13. 3D-echo confirmed the normalization of ejection fraction

Figures

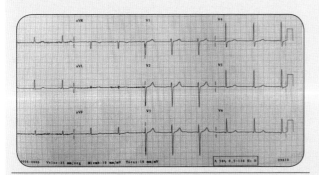

Figure 14.1. Baseline 12-lead electrocardiogram revealed a normal sinus rhythm with no associated conduction or repolarization abnormalities

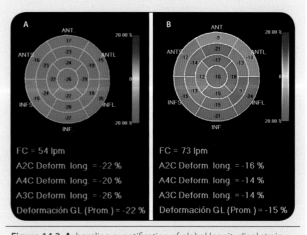

Figure 14.2. A: baseline quantification of global longitudinal strain in the normal range; B: after the third week of chemotherapy a significant fall in global longitudinal strain (GLS of -15%) was observed

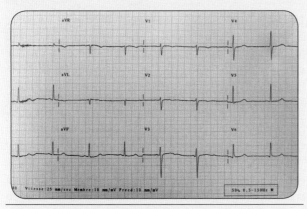

Figure 14.3. The 12-lead ECG at the end of the fifth cycle of chemotherapy revealed a long QT corrected interval (QTc of 553 ms)

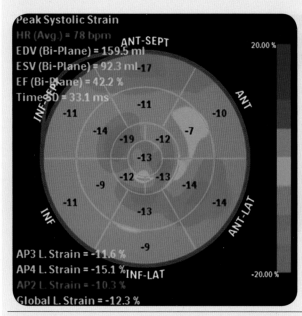

Figure 14.4. Significant decrease in GLS was observed after the fifth cycle of chemotherapy

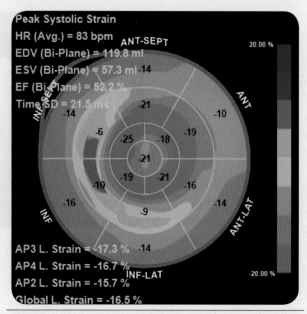

Figure 14.5. Post heart failure treatment we can see an improvement in deformation parameters (GLS -16.5%)

14.2. Discussion

Patients diagnosed with hematologic neoplasms, such as lymphoma or leukemia, are usually exposed to high-dose anthracyclines, which leads to a high-risk of drug-induced left ventricular dysfunction. Anthracyclines-induced cardiomyopathy has been studied in depth, being the chronic presentation the most frequently observed. Nevertheless, there have also been reports of acute and subacute toxicities (11% to 21% of cases), which are mainly related to a marked inflammatory response causing transient dysfunction of the cardiomyocytes.

This case is just one example of the daily dilemmas faced by both cardiologists and oncologists: What to do if a patient develops cardiotoxicity but otherwise has an aggressive tumor that requires the maintenance of anthracyclines? Former ASCO guidelines recommend the withdrawal of doxorubicin in patients who develop left ventricular dysfunction. However, there are no established guidelines or protocols that standardize treatment of subclinical ventricular dysfunction, detected with echo deformation parameters. Current studies include a small number of patients or are retrospective.

This decision is complex and should be individualized by means of a multidisciplinary team approach (mandatory nowadays). It

is essential to weigh the risk of anthracyclines withdraw, against the risk of ventricular dysfunction.

Early treatment of subclinical left ventricular dysfunction (in this case a significant > 15% decrease in global longitudinal strain, from baseline, in follow-up echocardiography) has been demonstrated to reduce the development of clinical left ventricular dysfunction. If we have a diagnosis of subclinical left ventricular dysfunction, and we need to continue with chemotherapy, an early cardioprotective regimen enables us to maintain oncologic treatment and to reduce cardiovascular adverse events.

Treatment with beta-blockers, ACEI, or aldosterone inhibitors, initiated in the early phase of left ventricular dysfunction, and maintained during follow-up increases the chances to improve, even under persistent exposure to the chemotherapy. There are no established guidelines or protocols that standardize normal values of the GLS, and even less on the therapeutic actions that should be taken if there is a considerable decline while a patient undergoes chemotherapy.

This case helps to prove the usefulness of deformation parameters as evidence of incipient myocardial damage, and should encourage maintaining a stricter echocardiographic follow-up or even the initiation of what should be considered secondary prevention drugs (beta-blockers, ACEI).

14.3. Conclusions

Cardiotoxicity associated with anthracyclines is frequently observed. If developed, an individualized and multidisciplinary approach weighing the risks and benefits of their withdrawal, and supporting the introduction of cardio-protective drugs (beta-blockers, ACEI, aldosterone antagonists) should be encouraged. Standardized protocols that include GLS for early detection of cardiotoxicity are desirable.

Case 15

Transtuzumab-Induced Cardiotoxicity

Alberto Cecconi
Carlos Ferrera Durán

Cardiology Department. San Carlos University Hospital. Madrid. Spain

15.1. Case Presentation

A 82-year-old male presented with a two-month history of fatigue and episodes of melena. He was diagnosed five years earlier with an aggressive CD20+ B-cell non-Hodgkin's gastric lymphoma and received six cycles of chemotherapy with rituximab, cyclophosphamide, doxorubicin, vincristine, and prednisolone that achieved a complete remission. As a collateral effect, the patient developed a peripheral neuropathy and an asymptomatic mild cardiac systolic dysfunction secondary to vincristine and anthracycline, respectively. Actually, he was just receiving treatment for hypertension.

During the evaluation of the bleeding, a gastroscopy led to diagnosing an HER2-positive advanced gastric adenocarcinoma located in the fundus. No metastasis was observed on the PET-

CT. Considering the age of the patient and the previous side effects of chemotherapy, the therapeutic strategy planned was complete resection surgery without neoadjuvant therapy. A total gastrectomy including spleen and greater omentum resection was performed.

A few months later a hepatic metastasis was documented and chemotherapy with capecitabine and trastuzumab started. Cardiotoxicity was monitored with intensive echocardiographic follow-up. Initially, the known mild cardiac systolic dysfunction was maintained stable **(Video 15.1)**, but six months later, although the patient had not developed any sign of heart failure, a progression to severe systolic dysfunction was detected **(Video 15.2 and Video 15.3)**. Consequently, trastuzumab was discontinued. Treatment with beta-blocker, ACEI and minerale-corticoid receptor antagonists was introduced. Three months later cardiac systolic function recovered to previous baseline **(Video 15.4 and Video 15.5)**.

Videos

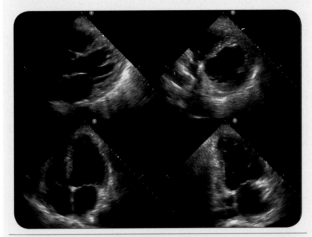

Video 15.1. Baseline echocardiography evaluation. Mild ventricular dysfunction (EF 48%) due to mild global hypokinesia

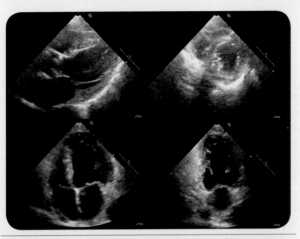

Video 15.2. Six months follow-up. Left ventricular function has clearly worsened after trastuzumab therapy (EF 31%)

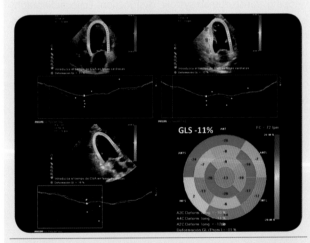

Video 15.3. Six months follow-up. Deformation study shows low GLS (-11%)

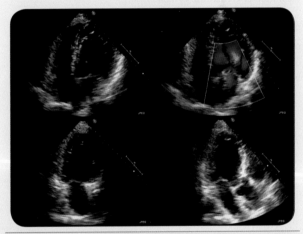

Video 15.4. Nine months follow-up. Cardiac systolic function recovered to previous baseline

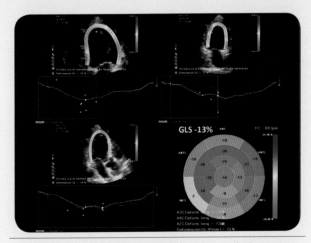

Video 15.5. Nine months follow-up. Deformation study shows a slight improvement in GLS (-13%)

15.2. Discussion

This case illustrates many of the features of cardiotoxicity secondary to trastuzumab. Trastuzumab is a monoclonal antibody against the human epidermal growth factor receptor-2 (HER2, also known as ErbB2). Its administration is approved for HER2-overexpressing metastatic gastric/gastroesophageal junction adenocarcinoma and for HER2-overexpressing breast cancer. However, HER2 is also a native cardiac protein and accumulation of anti-HER2 antibody in cardiomyocytes correlates with the occurrence of adverse side effects.

Trastuzumab-related cardiotoxicity is mainly expressed by an asymptomatic decrease in LVEF. The mechanism of alteration in contractility seems to be similar to stunning or hibernation. This hypothesis is supported by the absence of significant myocyte death in cardiac specimens and the usual recovery after drug discontinuation. Moreover, a new challenge is often tolerated after resolution of cardiac abnormalities.

Risk factors associated with cardiotoxicity include older age, previous or concurrent anthracycline use (especially if the cumulative doxorubicin dose is > 300 mg/m^2), pre-existing cardiac dysfunction, high body mass index, and antihypertensive therapy. No cumulative dose of trastuzumab correlates with cardiotoxicity.

Cardiac function should be assessed prior to commercing treatment and echocardiographic monitoring should be scheduled, especially in the adjuvant setting where a drug can be held or discontinued for asymptomatic cardiac dysfunction. In the metastatic setting, the clinical benefit provided by trastuzumab faces the risk of asymptomatic cardiac function decrease.

Although there is no specific study assessing the effects of standard treatment for cardiac systolic dysfunction in the specific scenario of trastuzumab-related cardiotoxicity, these patients should receive beta-blockers and ACEI.

15.3. Conclusions

The clinical history is the first step in the risk-stratification for developing transtuzumab-systolic dysfunction. Echocardiography is the most useful technique for cardiac monitoring and drug discontinuation often leads to a baseline recovery of cardiac function. In complex cases of metastatic disease, discontinuation of therapy is a complex decision that should weigh the echocardiography and clinical status against the potential benefit in the treatment of the oncologic disease.

Case 16

Shortness of Breath in a Hodgkin Lymphoma Patient

Susana del Prado Díaz
Zorba Blázquez Bermejo

Cardiology Department. La Paz University Hospital. IdiPAz Research Institute. Madrid. Spain

16.1. Case Presentation

A 74-year-old woman presented with fever and groin adenopathies. After a groin lymph node biopsy, she was diagnosed with nodular sclerosis Hodgkin lymphoma. The extension study evidenced IV-A stage with supra- and infra-diaphragmatic ganglionar, pleural, and bone involvement. Treatment was started with a PVAG regime (prednisolone, vinblastin, adriamycin, gemcitabine). After six cycles of the proposed scheme, a control positron emission tomography revealed reduced metabolic activity, with persistent FDG uptake of left scapula, clavicle, and left costal arches compatible with viable tumor. Pleura and left groin adenopathy also had an intense increase in FDG activity. After completing the treatment, the patient required a prolonged hospitalization due to herpetic encephalitis, complicated by epileptic seizures, although at discharge she barely presented any sequelae.

However, one month after discharge, the patient was admitted in the emergency room with progressive shortness of breath, orthopnea, and paroxysmal nocturnal dyspnoea. Shortly after admission, her condition worsened rapidly. Physical exam revealed hypotension, severe dyspnea, and cyanosis. New-onset atrial fibrillation with rapid ventricular response was observed on ECG **(Figure 16.1)** and her lab results showed respiratory insufficiency, pO_2 42 mmHg, and D-dimer of 9,812 µg/L (normal value < 500 µg/L).

An emergency echocardiography revealed a severely enlarged right ventricle with severe right ventricular dysfunction **(Video 16.1, Video 16.2, Video 16.3, and Video 16.4).** Right ventricle fractional shortening was 18%. Moderate tricuspid regurgitation enabled an estimation of systolic pulmonary artery pressure of 60 mmHg and inferior vena cava was dilated without respiratory variations. Left ventricle was hyperdynamic and no pericardial effusion was detected.

These findings strongly suggested a pulmonary embolism, but the patient was considered too unstable to undergo a computed tomography. Fibrinolysis was not performed because of high bleeding risk related to comorbidities and advanced age, so anticoagulation therapy and non-invasive mechanical ventilation were started. Although she initially required infusion of vasopressors due to significant hypotension, after 12 hours respiratory and hemodynamic stability was achieved and a computed tomography could be performed. It confirmed repletion defects in both main pulmonary arteries, consistent with a massive pulmonary embolism **(Figure 16.2).** RV/LV relation was > 1, suggesting right chamber pressure overload. A slight pleural bilateral effusion was detected. After 72 hours the patient was transferred to the cardiology ward. She was discharged 10 days later on low molecular-weight heparin with no oxygen therapy.

Videos

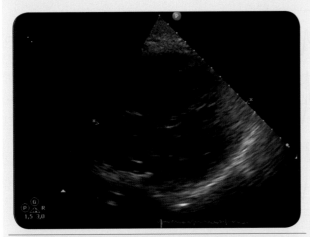

Video 16.1. 2D-echocardiography. The parasternal long-axis view shows an enlarged RV

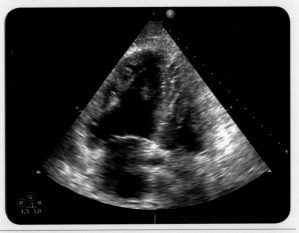

Video 16.2. 2D-echocardiography apical four-chamber view showing a severely enlarged and dysfunctional right ventricle. Ventricular septum is shifted towards the left ventricle

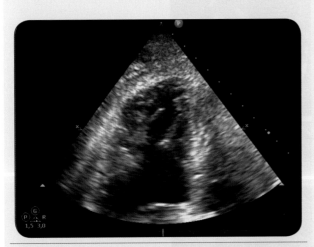

Video 16.3. 2D zoom of the right ventricle at the apical view. McConnell sign is present (regional pattern of right ventricular dysfunction, with akinesia of the mid free wall but normal motion at the apex)

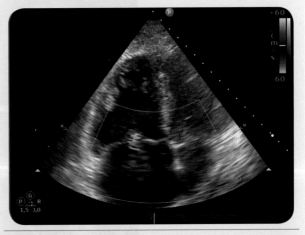

Video 16.4. Apical four-chamber view showing moderate tricuspid regurgitation

Figures

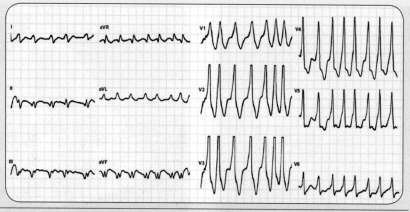

Figure 16.1. Electrocardiogram showing atrial fibrillation with rapid ventricular response

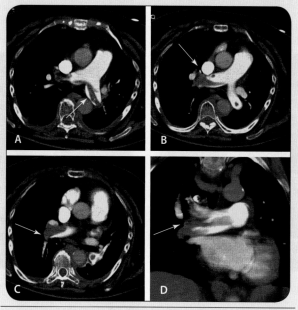

Figure 16.2. CT showing repletion defects in both main pulmonary arteries

16.2. Discussion

Cancer patients are at increased risk of thromboembolism. Pathogenesis seems to be multifactorial, involving local and systemic factors. Such events may result in considerable morbidity and impaired quality of life and, in some instances, may be life-threatening. Brain, ovary, pancreas, colon, stomach, lung, kidney, and liver cancers have the highest risk of deep vein thrombosis and pulmonary embolism; however, leukemia and lymphomas are also conditions prone to suffer thrombotic events.

Some anticancer drugs are associated with a higher risk of thrombotic events in addition to the risk of the tumor itself; among them we can include gemcitabine and vinblastin. Although the exact underlying mechanism is not completely understood, it is known that the combination of several of these drugs involves a higher thrombotic risk. Immobilization, age, presence of a central venous catheter, recent hospitalization, and high dose corticosteroid are also associated in this case with increased risk of pulmonary embolism.

In our case, the patient presented signs and symptoms consistent with an acute and massive pulmonary embolism. Although computed tomography angiography is the gold standard diagnostic imaging modality, sometimes hemodynamic instability limits its performance. Echocardiography, although insensitive for diagnosis, can play an important role in risk stratification and unstable patients, as it can be performed quickly as a bedside test. A normal echocardiography does not exclude a pulmonary embolism, but whenever a massive pulmonary embolism is suspected, we can expect a significant cardiac involvement. An enlarged and dysfunctional right ventricle strongly suggests pulmonary embolism, particularly when previous normal exams are available. McConnell sign is highly specific for pulmonary embolism. When pulmonary embolism is suspected anticoagulation therapy must be initiated straightaway, and after achieving hemodynamic stabilization, confirmed with computed tomography angiography.

16.3. Conclusions

Thrombotic phenomena are increased in cancer patients, and a variety of anticancer agents have been reported to increase the risk of thrombotic events. Early diagnosis and appropriate antithrombotic therapy are key to improve morbidity and mortality associated with pulmonary embolism.

Case 17

Right Atrial Mass in a Breast Cancer Patient

Zorba Blázquez Bermejo
Susana del Prado Díaz

Cardiology Department. La Paz University Hospital. IdiPAz Research Institute. Madrid. Spain

17.1. Case Presentation

A 44-year-old woman with past medical history of superficial thrombophlebitis was diagnosed with breast cancer after the performance of a biopsy from a palpable nodule. She was treated surgically with a right mastectomy and lymphadenectomy, the resected tumor being positive for hormonal receptors but negative for HER2. The extension study which consisted of a thoracic-abdominal-pelvic CT scan, bone scintigraphy, and tumor marker levels was negative.

Prior to beginning the chemotherapeutic regimen, a full evaluation was completed. The patient was clinically asymptomatic and the physical exam was normal. Blood tests revealed iron-deficiency anemia (Hb 10, 1 g/dL), as well as reactive thrombocytosis (598,000 platelets/μL). The chest X-ray revealed a port-a-cath placed in the right subclavian vein and the metallic component of the implanted tissue expansor. In the electrocardiogram normal sinus rhythm was confirmed with no associated conduction or repolarization abnormalities. At last, the echocardiographic parameters were within normal including an ejection fraction (65%) and a GLS of -20%.

The scheduled chemotherapeutic regimen included four cycles of adriamycin and cyclophosphamide, followed by four cycles of docetaxel. After the first month of active treatment, in the routine transthoracic echocardiography for the detection of cardiotoxicity, a 3 cm mass was detected in the right atrium. **(Video 17.1 and Video 17.2).** No contrast enhancement was seen after intravenous administration of a contrast agent **(Video 17.3).** Full mass characterization work-up comprised a transesophageal echocardiography which confirmed its dependence from the septal portion of the tricuspid valve without adhesion to the catheter **(Video 17.4).** A cardiac magnetic resonance was performed but the implanted tissue expansor made the images unsuitable for cardiac mass diagnosis.

Differential diagnosis included thrombus, infective endocarditis, and tumoral progression. As the patient remained afebrile and with negative infectious parameters on repeated blood tests, endocarditis did not seem probable. Nevertheless, erythema of the surrounding skin of the port-a-cath made microbiological sample testing obligatory, Staphylococcus aureus being isolated and, finally, the catheter removed with no additional established antibiotic treatment. Meanwhile, a therapeutic low molecular weight heparin regimen was initiated and complemented with close echocardiographic follow-up.

The mass had a progressive reduction, disappearing completely by the sixth week of the beginning of anticoagulation **(Video 17.5 and Video 17.6),** supporting the diagnosis of a thrombus. Pro-thrombotic states were ruled out and the patient completed the chemotherapeutic regimen with no other complications and with full remission of the primary tumor.

Videos

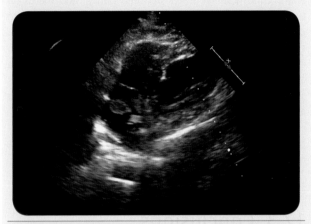

Video 17.1. Transthoracic echocardiography in parasternal view showing a mass of echo-lucent inside and extent mobility in the right atrium

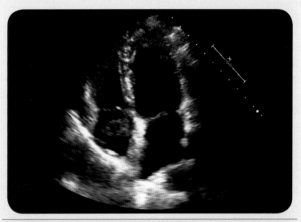

Video 17.2. Transthoracic echocardiography in apical four-chamber view demonstrating a mass of echo-lucent inside and extent mobility in the right atrium

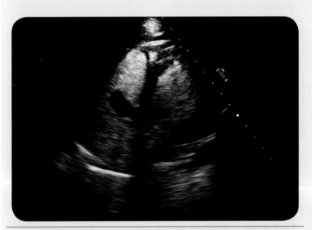

Video 17.3. Transthoracic echocardiography in parasternal view after administration of contrast agent that shows right atrial mass with peripheral contrast enhancement

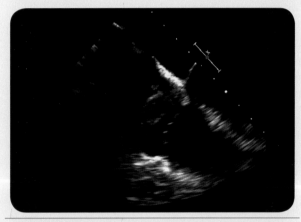

Video 17.4. Transesophageal echocardiography in midesophageal 0° four-chamber view showing right atrial mass depending on the septal portion of the tricuspid valve

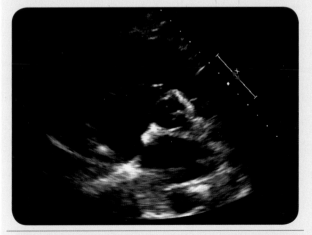

Video 17.5. Transthoracic echocardiography in parasternal short-axis view that demonstrates disappearance of right atrial mass

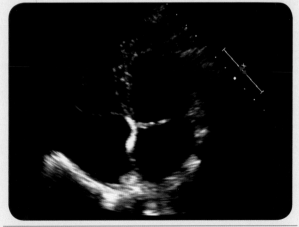

Video 17.6 Transthoracic echocardiography in apical four-chamber view showing disappearance of right atrial mass

17.2. Discussion

This clinical case supports the relevance of a standardized echocardiographic follow-up of oncologic patients who undergo chemotherapeutic regimens, not only for early detection of cardiotoxicity, but also because it can help identify other oncologic-derived complications. Cardiac masses are usually first detected at echocardiography. Nearly half the primary tumors in the right atrium are malignant and are predominantly found in males whereas most left atrial primary tumors are benign.

In oncologic patients, a pro-thrombotic state is favored not only by the tumor itself (released mediators), but also by its surrounding which includes sepsis (they are usually immunosuppressed patients), surgical interventions, thrombocytosis, central venous catheters, or specific pharmacologic agents (L-asparaginase, tamoxifen, estrogens, thalidomide analogs, cisplatin, and anti-angiogenic agents).

Differential diagnosis of intra-cardiac masses represents a true challenge in daily practice. Echocardiography is still the best choice for the initial diagnostic approach in this population, as it is not only accessible because of its low cost, but also because it offers a broad temporal resolution. Today, cardiac magnetic resonance imaging is the gold standard method for cardiac masses assessment. CMRI provides an advanced tissue characterization and accurately differentiates between benign and malignant tumors in a single examination. This assessment is important to plan therapy and to monitor tumor regression after surgery or chemotherapy. However, prosthesis artifacts decrease its feasibility. In these cases, transesophageal echocardiography can give additional information of the relationship of the mass with its surrounding structures and its functional behavior if a contrast agent is administered, as tumors with their high intrinsic vascularization tend to produce a marked and heterogeneous enhancement as opposed to thrombus which remains hypointense or with a slight peripheral enhancement.

17.3. Conclusions

Transthoracic echocardiography for the screening of oncologic patients who undergo treatments with cardiotoxic agents enables early detection of other associated life-threatening complications. Differential diagnosis of intracardiac masses is both complex and essential and may require the support of other imaging techniques such as transesophageal echocardiography with addition of contrast agents, CT or MRI.

Case 18

Secondary Cardiac Tumor after Osteosarcoma

Susana del Prado Díaz
Zorba Blázquez Bermejo

Cardiology Department. La Paz University Hospital. IdiPAz Research Institute. Madrid. Spain

18.1. Case Presentation

A 22-year-old man with a diagnosis of right knee osteosarcoma Broder grade 4, was treated with adjuvant chemotherapy with high dose methotrexate, cisplatin, adriamycin, and mifamurtide, followed by wide extraarticular resection. After one year, he was diagnosed with acute myeloid leukemia, probably secondary to previous anticancer treatment. An induction FLAG-IDA regimen and ARA-C (fludarabine, idarubicin, and cytarabine) consolidation was administered, with the intention of subsequently performing a bone marrow transplant. During the pre-transplant evaluation an echocardiography was performed, showing a normal left ventricle. The right ventricle also had normal size and function, but its refringence and thickness were increased, with a mobile mass attached to the ventricular surface of the tricuspid annulus (2.60 x 1.55 x 3.33 cm) **(Video 18.1, Video 18.2, Video 18.3, and Video 18.4).**

A cardiac magnetic resonance was performed to clarify the differential diagnosis between tumor mass and thrombus. It showed a mass with irregular edges and wide implantation base attached to the ventricular surface of the tricuspid valve and extension to the right ventricle anterior wall. It was isointense with the myocardium in T1- and T2-weighted sequences, and after gadolinium administration, it was partially perfused. Hypoperfused central areas corresponding to lack of late gadolinium enhancement were probably related to necrotic areas. These findings suggested tumoral etiology (osteosarcoma metastasis *versus* granulocytic sarcoma) **(Video 18.5 and Figure 18.1).**

A thoracic-abdominal-pelvis computed tomography excluded other distant metastases, and an ECG-gated cardiac computed tomography confirmed the presence of an heterogeneous attenuation mass arising from the tricuspid annulus and right ventricle free wall without pericardial extension **(Figure 18.2).** A transfemoral biopsy was performed under guidance with intracardiac echocardiography but, unfortunately, it failed to obtain a suitable sample from the mass. Metastatic disease from leukemia was the first suspicion, and an aggressive approach was attempted, performing a match-related allogenic bone marrow transplantation which was successful with a complication free course.

However, five months afterwards, a new computed tomography revealed pulmonary nodules and an echocardiography showed severe pericardial effusion, up to 3 cm at the left ventricle posterior wall, and a thickened visceral pericardium with irregular edges and filiform echodense mobile structures attached. Major echocardiographic signs of cardiac tamponade were not present. The mass had grown (67 mm) but did not cause obstruction of the tricuspid valve **(Video 18.6, Video 18.7, Video 18.8, and Video 18.9).** Large, echodense, left pleural effusion was observed, with filiform structures inside **(Figure 18.3).** Cytology from pleural effusion obtained by means of a thoracocentesis was consistent with metastatic progression of the patients osteosarcoma, and chemotherapy with carboplatin, etoposide, and ifosfamide was started.

However, six months afterwards, the patient was admitted with increasing dyspnea. A massive left pleural effusion with a new mass depending on the visceral pleura was discovered **(Video 18.10),** and computed tomography showed paraortic, pulmonary, pleural, and peritoneal progression of the disease. A new line of chemotherapy was started with gemcitabine-docetaxel, but his clinical status worsened and the patient finally died.

Videos

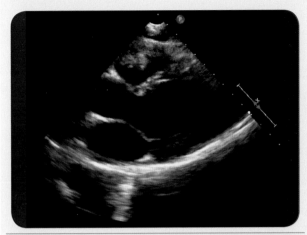

Video 18.1. Parasternal long-axis view showing a cardiac mass in the right ventricle inflow

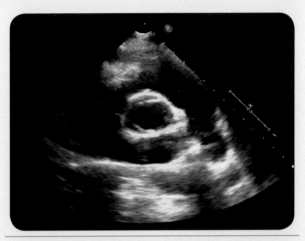

Video 18.2. Short-axis view at great vessels level showing a cardiac mass in the right ventricle inflow

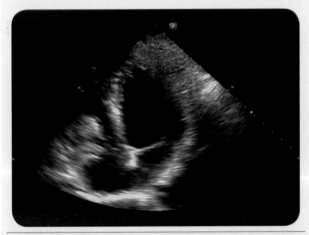

Video 18.3. Apical four-chamber view showing the mass attached to the ventricular surface of the tricuspid annulus

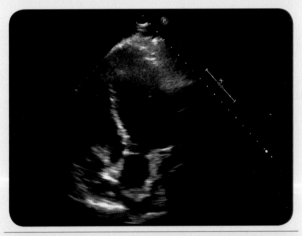

Video 18.4. Apical five-chamber view showing the mass attached to the ventricular surface of the tricuspid annulus

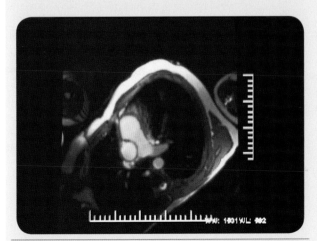

Video 18.5. Cardiac magnetic resonance, axial five-chamber SSFP cine sequence

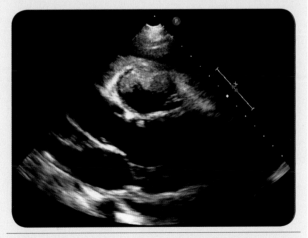

Video 18.6. Parasternal long-axis view showing the huge mass and pericardial effusion, with thickened visceral pericardium and echodense images attached to it in a "crown-like" fashion

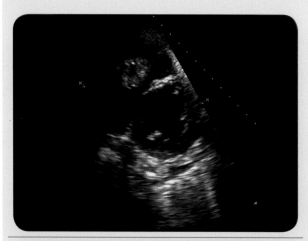

Video 18.7. Parasternal short-axis view. See **Video 18.6** for explanation

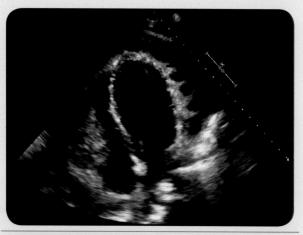

Video 18.8. Apical four-chamber view showing the cardiac mass and pericardial effusion

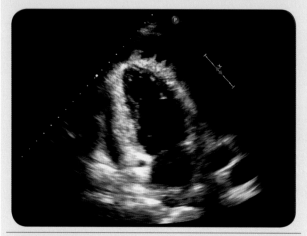

Video 18.9. Apical two-chamber view showing the cardiac mass and pericardial effusion

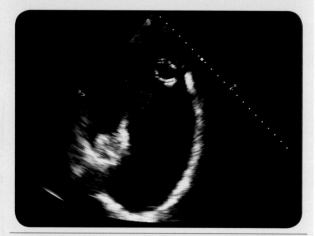

Video 18.10. Large pleural effusion. Metastatic mass attached to parietal pleura

Figures

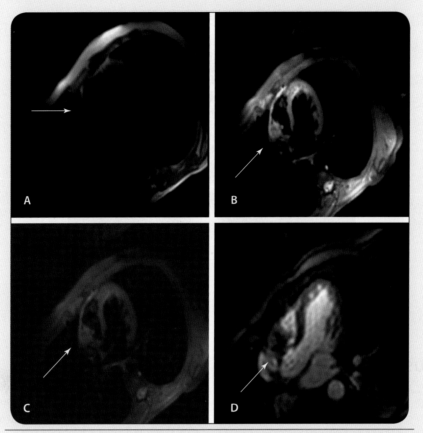

Figure 18.1. Cardiac magnetic resonance, long-axis images. Axial T1-weighted image **(A)**, double IR **(B)**, triple IR **(C)**, and T1-postcontrast image **(D)** showing heterogeneous late gadolinium enhancement, with central hypoperfused necrotic areas

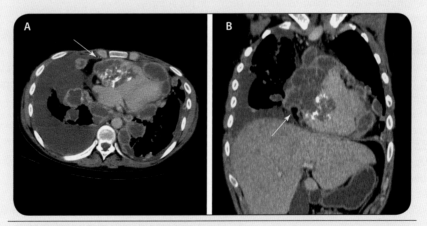

Figure 18.2. Computed tomography images showing heterogeneous attenuation mass arising from the tricuspid annulus without pericardial extension

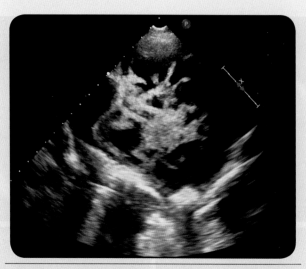

Figure 18.3. Large pleural effusion with filiform structures inside

18.2. Discussion

The finding of a new cardiac mass in a cancer patient always carries a complex differential diagnosis between secondary cardiac tumor or thrombus. Intracardiac biopsy can give us a definitive diagnosis, but it is often technically difficult, failing to obtain an adequate sample from the mass. Imaging techniques such as computed tomography or cardiac magnetic resonance can provide useful information regarding the etiology of the tumor. Cardiac magnetic resonance is the gold standard to evaluate cardiac masses, because of its potential for tissue characterization. Tumors present more frequently with heterogeneous late gadolinium enhancement and, typically, metastases have low signal intensity on T1-weighted images, and appear brighter on T2-weighted sequences. However, sometimes these findings are not consistent among the different tumors, and the appearance of thrombi varies depending on its evolution time. ECG-gated MDCT provides a higher spatial resolution, enabling better identification of the edges and potential infiltration of adjacent structures such as the pericardium.

In our case cardiac magnetic resonance and computed tomography suggested a tumoral etiology of the mass rather than a thrombus. However, it was still to be determined whether the mass derived from the acute myeloid leukemia (AML) or the osteosarcoma. Granulocytic sarcoma (chloroma) is a solid tumor composed of myeloblasts and is an infrequent manifestation of AML. On the other hand, ostesarcoma rarely metastasizes in the heart. When it happens, it usually occurs in the right ventricle outflow tract and the diagnosis is frequently made during the investigation for underlying causes of heart failure or, sometimes, in the autopsy.

The poor response to treatment was, in this case, the key to suspect the most likely etiology of the mass. As AML had a favorable evolution after bone marrow transplantation, metastatic osteosarcoma was the most reasonable option, later confirmed in pleural effusion pathology.

18.3. Conclusions

Differential diagnosis of intracardiac masses is sometimes challenging. Biopsy of the cardiac mass is not always feasible, and non-invasive imaging techniques can provide useful information regarding etiology and therapeutic and prognostic implications.

Case 19

Pulmonary Artery Sarcoma Mimicking a Pulmonary Embolism

Zorba Blázquez Bermejo
Susana del Prado Díaz

Cardiology Department. La Paz University Hospital. IdiPAz Research Institute. Madrid. Spain

19.1. Case Presentation

A 75-year-old man with a history of previous smoking habit, presented to the hospital complaining of two months of moderate exertional dyspnea. Upon physical examination a rude systolic murmur III/VI in the second left intercostal space and an attenuation of the intensity of the second heart sound were detected. The electrocardiogram was consistent with normal sinus rhythm at 60 bpm. On the chest X-ray there was evidence of widening of the superior mediastinum, as well as enlargement of the right heart cavities **(Figure 19.1)**. Transthoracic echocardiography revealed the presence an obstructive mass located in the main pulmonary artery and a markedly dilated and dysfunctional right ventricle **(Video 19.1 and Video 19.2)**.

As the main differential diagnosis included both massive pulmonary embolism and intravascular tumors, a magnetic resonance was performed in order to try to properly characterize the tissue. The reported size was 30 x 27 mm and it was located in both the main and right pulmonary arteries with a sub-occlusive behavior; the consistence was homogeneous, the imaging revealed low signal intensity on both T1- and T2-weighted sequences **(Figure 19.2)** and also important to note was its lack of late gadolinium enhancement. As the reported pattern is more frequently observed in thrombi rather than in tumors, the patient was diagnosed with pulmonary embolism and an anticoagulation regimen was established.

Clinical manifestations did not seem to improve and a control echocardiography confirmed the persistence of the mass. Hence, a CT scan was the chosen technique to complete the evaluation, ruling out the presence of segmental pulmonary embolism and associated pulmonary infarction **(Figure 19.3)**. CT scan suggested that the mass had its origin in the intravascular space itself.

Surgical removal was then scheduled, being complex and requiring reconstruction of the vascular walls with bovine pericardium. The surgical biopsy established the final diagnosis of pleomorphic sarcoma of the pulmonary artery. At first, the course seemed to be favorable with remission on further control echocardiographies **(Video 19.3)**. But after the second month of surgical intervention and complete exposure to adjuvant radiotherapy, a control CT scan detected not only local tumor relapse in the main pulmonary artery and mediastinal fat **(Figure 19.4)**, but also pulmonary metastatic disease. As it was now classified as a non-surgical tumor, a chemotherapeutic regimen with gemcitabine and dacarbazine was established, the initial response being incomplete and the patient having progressive asthenia, chest pain and edema in the low extremities. A new control CT scan revealed an increase in the size of the mass which now involved the left main and anterior descending coronary arteries **(Figure 19.5)**. Finally, a decision was made to pursue a palliative approach; the patient dying 10 months after diagnosis.

Videos

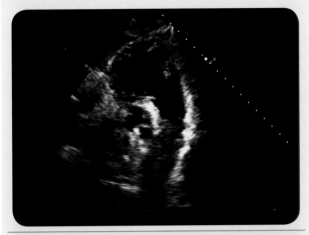

Video 19.1. Transthoracic echocardiography, short axis: obstructive mass in the main pulmonary artery

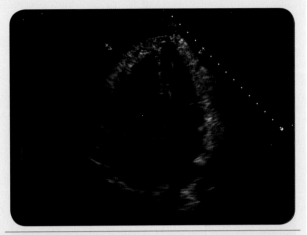

Video 19.2. Transthoracic echocardiography, apical four-chamber view: dilated and dysfunctional right ventricle

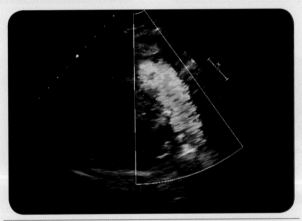

Video 19.3. Transthoracic echocardiography, parasternal short axis: postoperative echo study without residual mass in the main pulmonary artery and normal 2D Color Doppler pattern

Figures

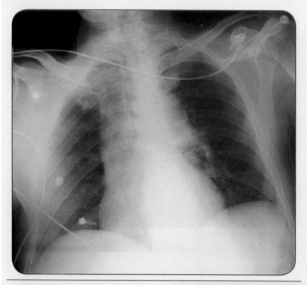

Figure 19.1. Posteroanterior chest X-ray: widening of the superior mediastinum and enlargement of the right cavities

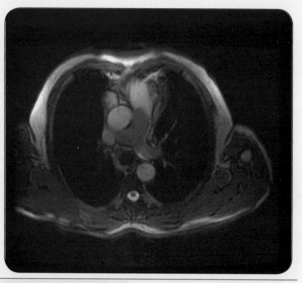

Figure 19.2. Short axis CINE magnetic resonance: hypointense mass in the main and right pulmonary artery with sub-occlusive behavior

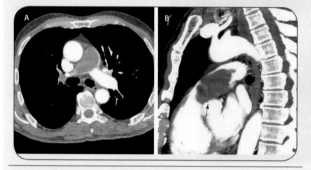

Figure 19.3. Contrast CT scan. **A:** intravascular mass within the main and right pulmonary artery. **B:** sagittal view of the CT scan: intravascular mass in the main pulmonary artery

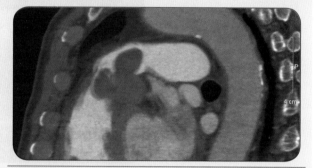

Figure 19.4. Contrast CT scan: lobulated mass in the main pulmonary artery that infiltrates its inferior wall, as well as the mediastinal fat

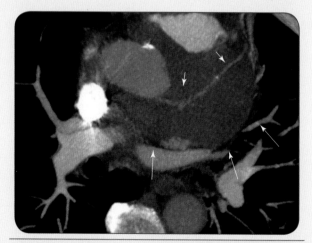

Figure 19.5. Sagittal view of the CT scan: the mass of the main pulmonary artery *(large arrows)* reaches the left main and anterior descending coronary arteries *(small arrows)* with reduction of their flow

19.2. Discussion

Angiosarcomas of the pulmonary artery are rare tumors with very unspecific clinical manifestations. In advanced stages, they may behave like a pulmonary embolism with symptoms derived mainly from flow obstruction or right ventricular dysfunction (heart failure). Symptoms may include dyspnea, chest pain, cough and hemoptysis. Its resemblance to pulmonary embolism often produces both a delay in diagnosis and inappropriate exposure to either anticoagulation or fibrinolysis. Failure to respond to such measures in addition to the absence of deep vein thrombosis, presence of anemia, weight loss or atypical images for a regular pulmonary embolism must arouse clinical suspicion.

The precise diagnosis of a cardiac mass after performance of routine imaging techniques might be uncertain. Nowadays, cardiac magnetic resonance plays an essential role in the differentiation of benign from malignant tumors, and especially tumors from thrombi with high accuracy. Some of the reported characteristics for malignant tumors include: larger sizes, heterogeneity and hyperintensity due to their intrinsic vascularization, extent mobility and, of course, the presence of late gadolinium enhancement. Nevertheless, tumors like angiosarcoma may have atypical behaviors on magnetic resonance due to their sometimes scarce vascularization that make them resemble thrombi patterns.

The treatment of this tumor is essentially surgical. There is a lack of large randomized studies analyzing the efficacy of chemotherapy or radiotherapy, but patients often undergo chemotherapy with a palliative intention. Prognosis relies on the success of full surgical removal; nevertheless, the overall long-term survival is still low. A series published in 2009 with 74 patients, showed a mean survival of 36.5 months if surgical intervention was performed *versus* 11 months when medical therapy was established.

19.3. Conclusions

Pulmonary artery angiosarcoma is a rare pathology that resembles a pulmonary embolism, situation that entails both a delay in diagnosis and exposure to inappropriate therapies. Directed cardiac magnetic resonance protocols may help with the differential diagnosis of tumor or thrombi. Surgical resection is the treatment of choice and complementary chemotherapeutic regimens are usually palliative. Even under the prelude of appropriate treatment, overall survival is very low.

Case 20

Atrial Fibrillation and Cancer

Carmen Olmos Blanco
Alberto Cecconi

Cardiology Department. San Carlos University Hospital. Madrid. Spain

20.1. Case Presentation

A 76-year-old female with personal history of right breast cancer in the past treated with chemotherapy (anthracyclines) and radical mastectomy 32 years ago revealed an invasive HER-2 positive ductal carcinoma of the left breast in a routine screening. After evaluation by the oncology team, the patient underwent tumorectomy (negative sentinel node and axillary infiltration), followed by adjuvant therapy with docexatel, carboplatin, and trastuzumab. Radiation therapy and hormone therapy with tamoxifen were subsequently initiated.

Shortly after beginning radiation therapy the patient started to complain of dyspnea and asthenia. Transthoracic echocardiography revealed normal biventricular function, with normal longitudinal strain values, and mildly enlarged left atrium **(Video 20.1, Video 20.2, and Figure 20.1).** The electrocardiogram demonstrated atrial fibrillation with rapid ventricular response. Bisoprolol, amiodarone, and oral anticoagulation therapy with acenocoumarol were then started. A few weeks later, the patient began to feel lightheaded and was admitted to the cardiology ward after she suffered two episodes of cardiogenic syncope. Physical exam was normal, and an electrocardiogram showed sinus bradycardia, with long QT interval (600 ms). A new echocardiography was performed, without significant changes compared to the previous study.

Bradycardia-inducing drugs were withheld, and 24-hour Holter monitoring performed five days after admission revealed sinus bradycardia, with two periods of atrial fibrillation with rapid ventricular response followed by long sinus pauses **(Figure 20.2).** The diagnosis of bradycardia-tachycardia syndrome was established, and she was referred for DDDR pacemaker implantation. Postoperative course was uneventful, and the patient was discharged from hospital, with good health condition in subsequent follow-up.

Videos

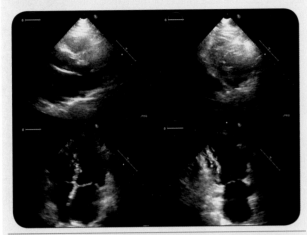

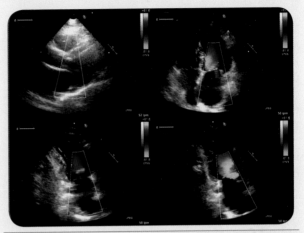

Video 20.1. 2D transthoracic echocardiography views showing normal LVEF and mildly dilated left atrium

Video 20.2. Color Doppler transthoracic echocardiography with normal intra-cardiac flows

Figures

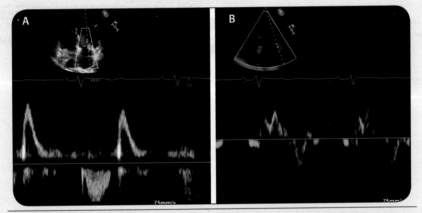

Figure 20.1. Pulsed wave Doppler across the mitral valve **(A)** and assessment of mitral annulus velocity by Doppler tissue imaging **(B),** showing normal E/A wave ratio, and E/E' ratio, both indicating no relevant diastolic dysfunction

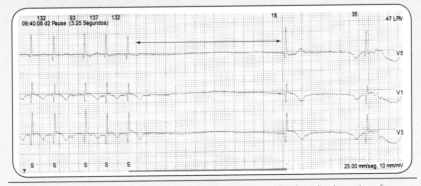

Figure 20.2. Holter monitoring showing a long pause and sinus bradycardia alternating after a burst of rapid atrial fibrillation

20.2. Discussion

The precise association between atrial fibrillation and cancer remains unknown. However, several studies have analyzed the incidence of new-onset atrial fibrillation after cancer surgery, particularly in lung cancer surgery, ranging between 6% and 32% in different series. Postoperative atrial fibrillation has been associated with poor prognosis, including increased post-operative mortality, prolonged hospital stay, and higher long-term mortality.

Factors predisposing to atrial fibrillation in cancer patients include advanced age, previous episodes of supraventricular arrhythmias, metabolic and electrolyte disorders, and increased sympathetic tone. In some cases atrial fibrillation might also represent a primary manifestation of the neoplasm (cardiac tumors or tumor of adjacent tissues). In addition, atrial fibrillation can be a consequence of chemotherapy. Different cytotoxic agents have been associated with a higher incidence of atrial fibrillation, including anthracyclines, cisplatin and carboplatin, 5-fluorouracil, paclitaxel and docetaxel, gemcitabine, ifosfamide, and supportive therapies such as corticosteroids, ondansetron and bisphosphonates. It has been proposed that the common pathway for these predisposing factors could be inflammation, although the complete underlying mechanisms are poorly understood.

In our case, the patient did not present any risks factors or previous structural heart disease, except mildly enlarged left atrium; however, she underwent breast tumorectomy and had been started on docetaxel and carboplatin, both associated with new-onset atrial fibrillation.

Although post-operative atrial fibrillation is a recognized entity, mainly in lung cancer patients, less is known about the relationship between chemotherapy and arrhythmias. In patients receiving these atrial fibrillation-inducing drugs, routine monitoring would be prudent. Among the parameters that could be employed to predict the risk of new-onset atrial fibrillation in cancer patients, natriuretic peptide levels and assessment of diastolic dysfunction by echocardiography could be useful.

Once atrial fibrillation is diagnosed, treatment must be focused on antithrombotic therapy and heart and rhythm control. Regarding anti-arrhythmic therapy, physicians should take into account possible side effects of these medications, such as QT interval prolongation, which may have an additive effect when used with common treatments in cancer patients, for example ondansetron or angiogenic inhibitors. Although radiofrequency catheter ablation has not been studied in depth in this population, it may be a reasonable alternative in patients with contraindications for rhythm control therapy or once this has failed.

The management of thromboembolic risk is particularly challenging in cancer patients. Malignancies involve high thrombotic risk, as cancer itself is a prothrombotic state; in addition, some drugs like novel angiogenic inhibitor have been associated with thromboembolic events. On the other hand, certain malignant neoplasias (hematologic cancer, brain tumors) carry an increased risk of severe hemorrhage. Therefore, initiation of antithrombotic therapy in cancer patients has to be strictly individualized, cautiously weighing the benefits against the risks according to the features of each patient.

Our patient had an infiltrative ductal breast carcinoma. This type of cancer does not entail a predisposition to bleeding, so in most cases anticoagulation therapy can be started without additional risk. In our case, after the initiation of beta-blockage therapy and amiodarone, significant sinus node dysfunction was documented, and pacemaker implantation was needed to achieve adequate rate control.

20.3. Conclusions

Atrial fibrillation has an increased incidence in patients with malignancies, particularly in those undergoing surgery, and it has been associated with poor prognosis. Factors associated with new-onset atrial fibrillation include comorbidities, antineoplastic agents and a pro-inflammatory state after surgery. Treatment of atrial fibrillation in cancer patients remains a challenge, particularly in terms of thromboembolic prevention, which must be individually tailored considering the risk/benefit ratio of each specific patient.

AUGMENTED REALITY

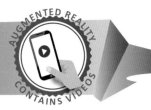

Our publications include Augmented Reality, which enables reproducing videos inside the book on an electronic device

① The first step is to download "JUNAIO" application onto your device. Both Apple and Android versions are available.

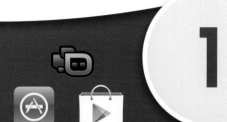

1

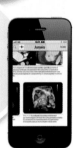

② Once downloaded, follow the instructions to visualize the videos inside the book.

1. Scan the cover of the book.
2. The channel that activates the videos will open.
3. Place the device over the image containing a video.
4. The video should activate on your device.

2

③ In case it does not work correctly by scanning the book cover, use the application´s search tool and enter the book title manually.

3

The video plays automatically on your electronic device

4

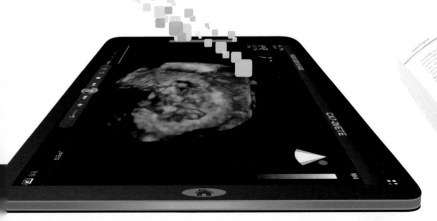

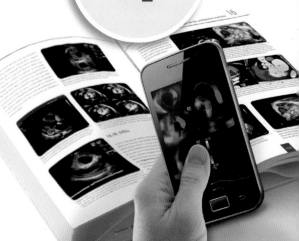